THE FAMILY AND PUBLIC POLICY

Frank F. Furstenberg, Jr., and Andrew J. Cherlin

GENERAL EDITORS

Stand by Me

The Risks and Rewards of Mentoring Today's Youth

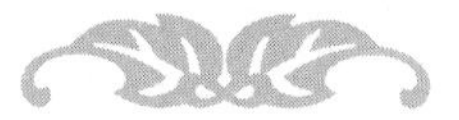

JEAN E. RHODES

Harvard University Press
Cambridge, Massachusetts
London England
2002

Printed in the United States of America

Library of Congress Cataloging-in-Publication Data

Rhodes, Jean E.
Stand by me : the risks and rewards of mentoring today's youth /
Jean E. Rhodes.
p. cm.—(The Family and public policy)
Includes index.
ISBN 0-674-00737-9 (alk. paper)
1. Socially handicapped youth—Services for—United States.
2. Social work with youth—United States.
3. Volunteer workers in social service—United States.
4. Mentoring—United States.
I. Title. II. Series.

HV1431 .R48 2002
362.79083—dc21 2001051856

For my mentor, George W. Albee

Contents

Stand by Me

Introduction

Youth mentoring programs are in the limelight. Over two million young people have a Big Brother, a Big Sister, or a similar adult volunteer involved in their lives, and the numbers are rising at an unprecedented rate. Although mentoring initiatives in the United States date back to the turn of the century, nearly half of all programs were established in the past five years, and only 18 percent have been operating for more than fifteen years.[1] And what we see today is just a beginning. Big Brothers Big Sisters of America—probably the best-known agency nationwide—has committed to doubling its size within five years, and other agencies have set similar goals.

This dramatic expansion in youth mentoring speaks volumes about the faith our society places in one-to-one relationships between vulnerable young people and nonrelated but caring adults. To help mentors bring about positive changes in the lives of their protégés (or mentees, as they are sometimes called), scores of organizations offer brochures, manuals, websites, toolkits, lists of best practices, and online advisors brimming with tips and detailed recommendations. The authority with which this information is presented often leads readers to conclude that most of the questions in the field have been answered.

Unfortunately, that is often not the case. These recommendations are rarely based on scientific research that has undergone peer review—not out of any intent to ignore findings or deceive readers but simply because such rigorous studies are in short supply. And it's not surprising, given how rapidly the youth mentoring phenomenon has grown, that few researchers have had a chance to step back and ask how—or, indeed, whether—these interventions help boys and girls navigate the rough shoals of adolescence. Today, despite the "buzz" surrounding the topic of mentoring, many important questions about the effectiveness of mentoring relationships remain unasked and unanswered. To explain what we currently know and to point out areas where our knowledge is still inadequate are my primary reasons for writing this book.

Stand by Me: The Risks and Rewards of Mentoring Today's Youth presents over a decade of my own research, as well as a synthesis of the findings of others. It is anchored in the ongoing work of Public/Private Venture (P/PV), a research, public policy, and program development organization. I cite several P/PV studies, but I give particular attention to their national evaluation of Big Brothers Big Sisters of America. This study is the largest, strongest, and the most influential evaluation of mentoring to date.[2] For the past several years, I have worked with Jean Baldwin Grossman, senior researcher at P/PV and co-author of the national evaluation, to further analyze the data from this study, with the goal of addressing basic questions about mentoring relationships. In synthesizing findings from these and other studies, my intention is not to add to the growing number of books that extol the virtues of mentoring but rather to bring some complexity and even some words of caution to the dialogue.[3]

From personal experiences, observations, and research, I am convinced of the extraordinary potential that exists within mentoring relationships. But I have also encountered the harm—rarely acknowledged—that unsuccessful relationships can do to vulnerable youth. One good relationship can transform a life, that's true; it can become the means by which a boy or girl connects with others, with teachers and schools, with their future prospects and potential. Yet because a close personal relationship is at the heart of mentoring, a careless approach can do tremendous damage to a child's sense of self and faith in others.

My strong contention—supported by findings that I will present in the following chapters—is that vulnerable children would be better left alone than paired with mentors who do not recognize and honor the enormous responsibility they have been given. Thus, instead of adding another voice to the chorus of calls for more and bigger mentoring programs, this book advocates a measured approach that builds on our growing knowledge about the risks, as well as the rewards, of mentoring. The goal of *Stand by Me* is to provide parents, policy makers, practitioners, and researchers with a deeper understanding of this very special human relationship and to assist them in making informed decisions about mentoring programs.

The Organization of This Book

A necessary starting point is a shared definition of the sometimes elusive word *mentor*. The term has generally been used in the human services field to describe a relationship between an older, more experienced adult and an unrelated, younger protégé—a relationship in which the adult provides ongoing guidance, instruction, and encouragement aimed at developing the competence and character of the protégé. Over the course of their time together, the mentor and protégé often develop a special bond of mutual commitment, respect, identification, and loyalty which facilitates the youth's transition into adulthood.[4] In this book, I will examine primarily relationships that take place within structured youth mentoring programs; though occasionally I will allude to other kinds of naturally occurring mentoring relationships, such as those between teachers and students or clergy and youth, they are not my central focus. Likewise, although group-mentoring, peer-mentoring, on-line mentoring, faith-based mentoring, and school-to-work apprenticeship programs are proliferating around the country, in the chapters that follow I will concentrate on in-person, one-to-one mentoring relationships between adult volunteers and youths. Eighty percent of the nation's programs match one mentor with one youth and thus fall within this category.[5]

In Chapter 1 I discuss some of the social and political factors that have ignited so much recent interest in mentoring, and I consider the sorts of evidence that can help us evaluate a program's effectiveness. This includes the national evaluation of Big Brothers Big Sisters mentioned above, as well as other programs.

In Chapter 2 I explore the underlying psychological processes by which volunteers bring about change. Previous theoretical work has emphasized the protective qualities of relationships between nonparent adults and vulnerable youth. According to this model, mentors increase the young person's resilience in the face of hardships, and therefore reduce the risk that the youth's development will take a negative turn. While compelling, the research supporting this model falls short of describing the actual mechanisms by which mentors bring about this increase in resilience. Similarly, this research sometimes fails to fully acknowledge the young person's ongoing relationships with parents and other adults who may have enormous influence on the course of development. The framework presented in this book places mentoring relationships within the broader cultural contexts of adolescents' lives.

Among the many things that change as adolescents grow and mature is the way they think about relationships. It should come as no surprise, then, that the benefits of mentoring accrue over a relatively long period of time. Earlier-than-expected terminations that dissolve the bond of trust between mentor and protégé appear to touch on vulnerabilities in youth in ways that other, less personal programs do not. In Chapter 3 I describe a mentoring bond that failed, in order to highlight both the benefits of enduring relationships and the potentially harmful effects on youths when mentors fail to deliver consistent support. Many programs take a rather cavalier approach to relationships between mentors and protégés, treating them as though the actual people involved are interchangeable. If one mentor doesn't work out, according to this view, another one can be quickly substituted, with no permanent harm done. I offer explanations for this misdirected thinking on the part of some program directors about the uniqueness of a given relationship. These explanations include our culture's tendency to equate healthy development with growing independence and therefore to devalue relationships over the life span, as well as developmentalists' emphasis on infant bonding with the mother. Both of these philosophical stances minimize the range of relationships, both good and bad, that shape developmental outcomes throughout life, not just in childhood.

Every year, caseworkers pair thousands of mentors with youth, based in part on guidelines from organizations like The National Mentoring Partnership, but mostly based on their own experience and intuition about the "fit" of particular mentors with particular youth. No rigid guidelines should ever replace the judgment, experience, and flexibility that real human beings bring to this very human activity. Nonetheless, the initial process of match-making, and the ongoing guidance that case workers offer mentors, youths, and their parents, could benefit from the rich research literature that has already been compiled on other helping relationships, particularly psychotherapy and interpersonal relations. Chapter 4 will highlight some of the lessons from emotional and behavioral therapy that might be profitably applied to the mentoring relationship.

In Chapter 5, I ask how programs might better respond to the developmental needs of youth, and I make recommendations for research and policy priorities. A continuing challenge will be to conduct more fine-grained evaluations that can decipher which program features, mentor styles, and relationship characteristics are most influential, and then to use that knowledge to make adjustments in existing programs. Evaluations that try to determine specific mentor characteristics that lead to the longest-duration relationships could have immediate and practical benefits for youth.

Although all adolescents in Western society are likely to share certain developmental processes, their unique circumstances, cultures, and identities often shape the meaning and quality of mentoring relationships. Many different aspects of identity intersect with one another in complicated ways during the formative teen years. Throughout the book, I discuss some of the sensitivities that emerge within subgroups of adolescents around issues of gender, ethnicity, race, and class, and the impact of these factors on the mentoring relationship.

Mentoring by volunteers is not a panacea, and it is not as inexpensive a public policy initiative as it may seem at first glance. Mentoring programs for vulnerable youth cannot substitute for a caring community of support, or for adequate public investment in adolescents' education, physical health and safety, and psychological well-being. Nonetheless, mentoring programs have proven that they can powerfully influence positive development among youth, and I believe that their careful expansion is warranted. Our challenge is, first, to not underestimate the complexities of mentoring relationships and, second, to better understand and promote the conditions under which they are most likely to flourish.

1

Inventing a Promising Future

> She gathers me. The pieces that I am, she gathers them and gives them back to me in all the right order.
>
> Toni Morrison, *Beloved*

On a warm May evening, seventh-grade teacher Nancy Jamison stood before a group of volunteer mentors and youth at an awards ceremony to introduce her protégé, Angela Hall. "Angela was a student in my health class five years ago and you might say that she and I just clicked," she said, smiling warmly in the direction of a young woman seated nearby. "I never had a daughter of my own," continued the 53-year-old teacher, "so when my sons and I did things, we'd always include Angela." When Nancy heard about a local mentoring initiative, in which modest college stipends were awarded to youths who remained in the program, she chose to formalize her relationship with Angela. "Besides," she laughed, "it gave me a built-in excuse to see her. I am deeply grateful for that." Next, Angela took the podium and described her academic successes, including a recently awarded college scholarship. What neither she nor Nancy mentioned that evening was that the seventh grader with whom Nancy had "clicked" five years earlier had recently lost her mother to murder and was living in a neighborhood where virtually all of her classmates were succumbing to the stresses of urban poverty.

Most of us know of instances in which a special bond enabled a child or adolescent to overcome even the most horrific life circumstances. Such stories tend to touch us deeply and restore our belief in the healing power of human connection. In Angela's case, the benefits were quite clear. Although her three younger siblings were struggling with academic and behavioral problems, Angela graduated early from high school and has maintained a B+ grade-point average in college.

Her successes did not come easily. Nancy provided Angela with the encouragement and direction that she needed to get through high school. When Angela resolved, on several occasions, to quit a summer college preparatory program, Nancy shored her up with love, tutoring, and reminders of the scholarships that lay ahead. In eleventh grade, when Angela received a five-day suspension for getting into a fistfight, Nancy provided coaching on anger control and worked with Angela through missed course material and homework assignments. Nancy also guided her through the college selection and application process and, when Angela's SAT scores came in low, worked with her to bring them up. Currently, Nancy exchanges regular emails with Angela at college, always ending them with the same advice: "Remember what you're there for."

Angela's story fits with research literature that has emerged from various fields, all of which suggests that supportive older adults, whether teachers, neighbors, extended family members or volunteers, contribute to positive outcomes for youth who are living in high-risk settings.[1] In their classic study *Growing Up Poor*, the sociologists Terry Williams and William Kornblum concluded that a key difference between successful and unsuccessful youth from lower-income urban communities was mentoring—the successful ones had mentors, the unsuccessful ones did not. They write, "The probabilities that teenagers will end up on the corner or in a stable job are conditioned by a great many features of life in their communities.

Of these, we believe the most significant is the presence or absence of adult mentors."[2] Similarly, the sociologist Bernard Lefkowitz recognized supportive adults as a vital protective influence on at-risk youth. Among the low-income adolescents he studied, "Again and again, I found that the same pattern was repeated: the kid who managed to climb out of the morass of poverty and social pathology was the kid who found somebody, usually in school, sometimes outside, who helped them invent a promising future."[3]

Such intergenerational relationships have long been recognized as an important resource in African-American communities.[4] Patricia Collins described the protective influence of "othermothers" in the African-American community—women who provide guidance to younger members of the community, often acting as surrogate parents and creating an "ethic of caring" among African-American women for one another's children.[5] Support networks often include other "fictive" kin—unrelated people who have been absorbed into an existing family structure as aunts, uncles, cousins, and siblings.[6] Many Latino families are also embedded in extended kinship networks that include not just blood relatives but other important adults as well.[7]

Nearly forty years ago, the psychiatrist Gerald Caplan discussed the psychological benefits of intimate, nonprofessional caregivers or "extrafamilial helping figures . . . such as older people with a reputation for wisdom."[8] He argued that such people are much closer to the individuals in need, both "geographically and sociologically," than professional caregivers. They occupy a position between the latter and the family member and are generally far more likely than the professional to be called on for support. Particularly in low-income communities, such informal caregivers are the prime sources of help when personal troubles develop.[9]

In a more recent survey of 294 adolescents, Sharon Beier and colleagues found that those with natural mentors were significantly less likely to participate in four of five high-risk behaviors they measured: smoking, drug use, carrying a weapon, and unsafe sex. Participation in the fifth high-risk behavior, alcohol use, was not affected.[10] Similarly, in a survey of 770 low-income urban adolescents, Marc Zimmerman and colleagues found that those with natural mentors had more positive attitudes toward school and were less likely to use alcohol, smoke marijuana, and become delinquent.[11] Additionally, my colleagues and I have found a consistent pattern of positive mentor influence in the lives of pregnant and parenting adolescent girls. The teenagers with natural mentors exhibited lower levels of alcohol consumption during pregnancy, better psychological functioning, and better vocational and educational outcomes than those without such supports.[12]

The Loss of Adult Support

Unfortunately, many youth do not readily find older, supportive adults beyond the boundaries of their household. Shifting marital patterns, overcrowded schools, and loss of community cohesiveness have dramatically reduced the availability of caring adults and restricted their opportunities for informal contact with youth.[13] The social fabric is stretched particularly thin in urban centers. Manufacturing jobs that once offered families economic stability and supported conventional values have given way to low-paying service jobs and unemployment. Many of the middle-class adults who once served as respected authority figures in the community have fled to the suburbs,[14] and far fewer of the adults who remain are willing or able to offer support and guidance to youth outside their families. Too often, adolescents turn to drug dealers and gang leaders for a sense of identity, purpose, and belonging.[15] Adults recognize the importance of close, one-to-one relationships with youth; the problem they face is a lack of time and opportunity. According to a recent Gallup poll, 75 percent of adults reported that it is "very important" to have meaningful conversations with children and youth, yet fewer than 35 percent reported actually having such conversations.[16]

The expansion of professional human services over the past thirty years has also stifled the growth of informal mentoring relationships.[17] Professionalization in these fields has led many adults to doubt their "common capacity to care" and to withhold guidance and support because of a mistaken belief that the social services sector will design intervention programs to take up the slack.[18]

The entry of more and more women into the workforce over the past thirty years has changed the landscape of American families, and a public response to these changes has lagged. Schools operate in a time warp, oblivious to the fact that 80 percent of their students now have working mothers. In many areas, schools offer kids few alternatives to hanging out on street corners or staying in unsupervised homes each afternoon. For months during the summer, schools literally close their doors to this very serious demographic reality. Fewer parents, particularly mothers, are now available to provide transportation or serve as leaders in after-school programs. Within single-parent families and other low-income households, the demands of growing children coupled with inflexible work schedules translate into even more constrained choices for youths. Middle-class, two-parent, suburban families, on the other hand, tend to schedule children into a dizzying array of disconnected music lessons, sports, clubs, and other structured activities that leave little time for family dinners, let alone informal interactions with adults.

Burgeoning class sizes have resulted in fewer teachers per student and fewer opportunities for the sorts of school-sponsored extracurricular activities that give rise to informal connections between youth and committed teachers, coaches, and counselors. The extracurricular activities that do exist within communities have become increasingly age-segregated, further limiting opportunities for intergenerational contact.[19] Many adolescents fill their non-school hours with part-time jobs, working under supervisors who are not much older than themselves.[20] Still other adolescents spend their non-school hours in unstructured and unsupervised situations.[21] Although policy makers are beginning to address the need of adolescents for adult supervision, this response has not kept pace with demand. The only public response to out-of-school needs—a patchwork of unevenly distributed programs with underpaid, highly mobile staff—is scandalously insufficient.

To some extent, middle-class parents have purchased adult contact and protection for their children through investment in after-school programs, sitters, athletic clubs, music lessons, summer camps, and even psychotherapy. For the 20 percent of adolescents who live in poverty and do not have these options for supervision, the loss of adult helpers within the community is much more threatening. But all youth are experiencing fewer opportunities for informal adult contact than they did in the past. Indeed, Laurence Steinberg has observed that few adolescents have even one significant, close relationship with an adult outside the family prior to reaching adulthood.[22]

When peers fill this vacuum, as they so often do in the adsence of adults, problems easily arise. Juvenile arrests almost doubled during the 1980s and 1990s, and the homicide rate for youths aged 14 to 17 nearly tripled.[23] As the Carnegie Council on Adolescent Development observed over a decade ago: "Many young people feel a desperate sense of isolation. Surrounded only by their equally confused peers, too many make poor decisions with harmful or lethal consequences."[24]

Can Volunteer Mentoring Fill the Gap?

To address the needs of youth who lack attention from caring adults, people from a wide spectrum of disciplines and interests are turning to volunteer mentoring programs. Whether the problem on the table is welfare reform, education, violence prevention, school-to-work transition, or national service, mentoring is mentioned again and again as the panacea.[25]

The mentoring approach is not new. Its roots can be traced to the Friendly Visiting campaigns of the late nineteenth century, which arose in American cities in response to what reformers perceived of as a widening gap between the rich and poor. In these volunteer programs, middle-class women attempted to form personal relationships with children in poverty. Although that particular movement eventually lost steam, the interest of the middle class in improving poor children's lives through volunteer work continued into the twentieth century.[26]

The most prominent organization to arise from that interest was Big Brothers Big Sisters of America. Beginning in the early 1900s, individual agencies were founded in various cities, and since that time over a million children have been matched with volunteers through more than 500 agencies in all fifty states. Outside of this organization, more than 4,500 other active mentoring initiatives have been established at the local, state, and national level.[27]

Although most local and state efforts are decentralized, a growing array of umbrella organizations—such as The National Mentoring Partnership, Mentoring USA, America's

Promise, and Connect America—have brought visibility, coherence, and momentum to the movement. The National Mentoring Partnership, an advocacy organization that provides materials and training to mentoring programs, has vigorously promoted the concept of "bringing mentoring to scale" and has developed an infrastructure of programs at the state and local level. Its website, www.mentoring.org, receives two million visits per month.[28]

Why Mentoring?

Public awareness of the difficult circumstances of disadvantaged youth and media attention to the importance of adult involvement account for much of the recent growth of mentoring programs. This growth also reflects a sense of disconnection from civic and family life that many middle-class adults feel and wish to remedy.[29] Unlike other forms of civic engagement, which are waning, volunteer mentoring is on the rise. Robert Putnam attributes this fact to the decentralized nature of the enterprise, which can accommodate the busy schedules of working adults and the physical constraints of older volunteers.[30] Another factor is a growing awareness within communities that problems among youth most often occur during unsupervised hours after school. Welfare reform, which moved poor single mothers into the labor force, has put additional pressure on the few supervised after-school programs that exist for low-income school-aged children and has made community leaders more appreciative of the relief that mentoring programs can provide.[31]

Concurrent with these trends, researchers and practitioners have shifted their attention from the prevention of specific disorders to a more general focus on positive aspects of youth development.[32] This has led to heightened interest in youth programs. Organizations such as the YMCA, Boys and Girls Clubs of America, and Big Brothers Big Sisters, which all have long histories, have recently come under the close scrutiny of researchers who adhere to an emerging youth-development philosophy.[33] Instead of focusing on problems, these researchers have attempted to identify "developmental assets," which are competencies and resources within young people's lives that enhance their chances of positive development.

In a national survey of youth, the Minnesota-based Search Institute found that the greater the number of such developmental assets present in a youth's life, the lower the rate of risk-taking behaviors. These researchers created a list of forty assets that are conducive to adolescents' healthy development, including "support from three or more other adults" and "adult role models."[34] Along similar lines, Shepherd Zeldin and colleagues reviewed more than 200 research studies and concluded that, in order to successfully pass through adolescence, youth need "access to safe places, challenging experiences, and caring people on a daily basis."[35] Mentoring is often seen as an important avenue for fulfilling these needs.

Evaluation of Mentoring

Despite the glow that surrounds mentoring, only a handful of research studies on the topic have been published in academic journals, and methodological shortcomings have clouded interpretations of those findings. Few studies have included comparison groups, statistical controls, or follow-up evaluations. Many studies report only correlations, making it difficult to disentangle cause from effect. For example, the finding that mentoring relationships go hand in hand with healthy, better-adjusted youth could be explained by the fact that well-adjusted youth are often more appealing to, and sought out by, adults and thus more likely to form mentoring relationships. And because mentoring programs are often components of larger youth programs, isolating their specific influence is extremely difficult.

These kinds of problems in the design of the few studies we have, combined with an abundance of anecdotal claims, have created considerable confusion about whether mentoring actually brings about the positive results that are so often hyped in the media. Nonetheless, a small but growing number of well-executed studies are converging to suggest that mentoring programs can have positive emotional, behavioral, and academic effects.[36]

The evaluation of Big Brothers Big Sisters of America by researchers at Public/Private Ventures in Philadelphia is perhaps the most influential study of mentoring to date. Many of the findings presented in the following chapters were based on data derived from this national study, whose participants, methods, and findings I describe below.[37]

The National Evaluation of Big Brothers Big Sisters

This study included 1,138 youth, all of whom applied to one of eight Big Brothers Big Sisters programs in 1992 and 1993. Boys represented slightly more than half of the sample, and approximately half of the youth were members of minority groups. Participants ranged in age from 10 to 16. Ninety percent of the participants lived with one parent—in most cases, their mother—and more than 40 percent lived in households that were receiving public assistance of some kind.

Youth were randomly assigned either to the group who would receive mentors (the treatment group) or to the group on the eighteen-month wait list. Initial questionnaires were given immediately after random assignment but before youth were told whether they were in the treatment or control group. The questionnaires were anonymous and confidential, and identification numbers on the forms were used to match students' answers over time without revealing their names. The initial questionnaire included questions about problem behavior, academic achievement, family relationships, peer relationships, and self-image.[38] Additionally, caseworkers, parents, and youth shared their impressions of the mentoring relationships. At the study's outset, the only difference between the treatment and control groups was that youth in the treatment group had the opportunity to be matched immediately with mentors.

Agency staff matched particular adult volunteers with particular youth on the basis of gender (only same-sex matches) and a variety of factors, including shared interests, reasonable geographic proximity, and, in some instances, race. At the conclusion of the study, 378 (78 percent) of youth in the treatment group had been matched.[39] The matches met for an average of eleven months, with more than 70 percent meeting at least three times a month.

After eighteen months, the two groups were given the questionnaires a second time and compared on a number of points. Although youth in *both* groups showed increases in academic, social-emotional, behavioral, and relationship problems over this period of time, the problems of the youth in the group that received mentoring increased at a slower rate. They also reported higher levels of functioning on several items and scales than did youth on the wait list: fewer days of class skipped, lower levels of substance use, less physical aggression, more positive parent and peer relationships, and higher scholastic competence and grades.

This pattern of findings held for boys and girls across race. Within-race comparisons yielded additional findings. In particular, minority girls in the group that received mentoring reported higher scholastic competence than minority girls in the control group. Similarly, minority boys in the group that received mentoring felt more emotionally supported by their peers than minority boys in the control group and were less likely to report that they had started to use drugs.[40]

On Second Glance

But just how big were these differences in benefits? In statistical terms, *effect size* represents the degree to which two groups differ (for example, the mentoring group versus the wait-listed group) and hints at the practical importance, as opposed to simply the statistical significance, of a finding. Although there are no easy conventions for determining practical importance, an effect size of around .20 is generally considered to be small, .50 is considered moderate, and .80 is considered large.[41]

DuBois and colleagues calculated two different effect sizes from the Big Brothers Big Sisters data: the magnitude of change over time (pre-program versus post-program estimates) and the post-program difference between participants in the mentoring versus the wait-listed groups. Average pre- versus post-program and group difference effect size estimates were low (.02 and .05, respectively), a finding "not necessarily consistent with the manner in which results of the large-scale evaluation frequently have been cited by the media as demonstrating a large impact for mentoring relationships."[42]

This inconsistency can be understood when we consider that *all* of the youth, including those who had mentors, showed gradual increases in problems over time. The youth who met with mentors worsened at a slower rate than control youth, but this is not the same as improving. Subsequent summaries of the study appearing on websites, in program materials, and in the literature often claim that the participants were less likely to use illegal drugs, less likely to skip school, and so forth, without qualifying that these differences were in comparison to a control group and *not* in comparison with their own behavior at the beginning of the program. All youths showed a greater likelihood of problem behaviors over the course of the eighteen-month period.

Even when accurately qualified, however, these findings are promising. Problem behaviors, relationship instability, and feelings of inadequacy are hallmarks of adolescence that tend to increase over time among teenagers, until they taper off by the early twenties.[43] The fact that a mentoring program was able to attenuate some of these destructive but developmentally normal behaviors across diverse relationships and youth is laudable and gives grounds for cautious optimism about the viability of the mentoring approach. But in light of the vast continuum in the quality and duration of mentoring relationships, no program could be expected to produce, within a relatively short time, dramatic, across-the-board reversals of the negative trajectories typical of adolescence.

The truth of the matter is that the mentor-protégé matches made by Big Brothers Big Sisters—and presumably those made through other programs as well—vary considerably in their effectiveness, depending on the characteristics of the individuals involved and the quality of the relationships they form. When Jean Grossman and I reanalyzed the Big Brothers Big Sisters data taking the quality and length of relationships into account, wide variations in program effects emerged.[44] But when all adolescents are combined, as was the case in the national evaluation, positive outcomes are easily masked by the neutral and even negative outcomes associated with less effective relationships.

Do these modest, and sometimes even negative, effects

mean that we should abandon mentoring as an intervention strategy? Of course not—but it does suggest that we should be more prudent in our claims, acknowledging the enormous variability across and within programs. The challenge is to distinguish between effective and ineffective relationships and to understand the contexts that give rise to each.

Analyzing the Effects of Mentoring Programs

In an attempt to do just that, DuBois and colleagues used a research technique called meta-analysis to review 55 evaluations of youth mentoring programs, including the Big Brothers Big Sisters study.[45] Meta-analysis permits researchers to synthesize the results of numerous studies on a single topic and to statistically determine the strength and consistency of program-related effects.

The researchers began by identifying all of the relevant studies on the topic of mentoring. To be included in the analyses, studies had to meet several criteria. First, the evaluated program needed to include a one-to-one relationship in which an older, more experienced mentor was paired with a younger (under 19) protégé. Second, the study had to examine empirically the effects of participation in a mentoring program, by pre-program versus post-program comparisons of the same group of youth or by comparisons between one group of youth receiving mentoring and another group not receiving mentoring. After identifying relevant studies, the researchers summarized the results of each study and then calculated effect sizes across the entire group of studies.

The favorable effects of mentoring programs were found to hold true across relatively diverse types of program samples, including programs in which mentoring was provided alone or in conjunction with other services. The positive effects were found both in programs that had general goals and in those with more focused goals. The positive effects held up for youth of varying backgrounds and demographic characteristics. Among the minority of studies that included follow-up assessments, the benefits of mentoring appeared to extend a year or more beyond the end of a youth's participation in the program.

As DuBois and colleagues note, however, the magnitude of these effects on the average youth participating in a mentoring program was quite modest.[46] Although there was considerable variation across studies, the average effect size across the samples was relatively small (.13), particularly in comparison to the effect sizes that have been found in meta-analyses of other mental health prevention programs for children and adolescents (such as .34 for Outward Bound).[47]

But while the overall effect size was modest, substantial variation in the effectiveness of different programs showed up across these studies. First, in programs where youth had more favorable life circumstances and better psychological and social functioning at the onset, effect sizes were larger. Strong effects also emerged for those youth who had more frequent contact with their mentors, who felt some emotional closeness to them, and whose mentoring relationships lasted longer. Program practices that ensured longevity—by providing training for mentors, offering structured activities for mentors and youth, having high expectations for frequency of contact, enjoying greater support and involvement from parents, and monitoring overall program implementation—led to stronger effects.

These practices, which speak to the adequacy of a program's infrastructure, converge with those identified by other researchers.[48] Sipe, for example, in a review of the literature, found three features that are essential to the success of any mentoring program: (1) screening, (2) orientation and training, and (3) support and supervision.[49] When one or more of these features was missing from a program, it had greater difficulty sustaining mentor-protégé relationships.

In the chapters that follow, I will return to these themes and suggest ways that programs might better address the needs of youth.

2

How Successful Mentoring Works

> "Why did you do all this for me?" [Wilbur] asked. "I don't deserve it. I've never done anything for you." "You have been my friend," replied Charlotte. "By helping you, perhaps I was trying to lift my life a trifle. Heaven knows, anyone's life can stand a little of that."
>
> E. B. White, *Charlotte's Web*

Patrick Summers walked through the crowded hallways of his middle school like a seasoned politician, gesturing confidently to his classmates and friends. With shoulders that advertised hours of weightlifting and wrestling practice, Patrick seemed to own the place. Not bad for someone who, only ten months earlier, had been on the brink of expulsion from school for a pattern of fighting. The worst incidents had broken out in his trailer park, shortly after he and his older brother had witnessed one of his mother's boyfriends physically abuse her. According to Patrick, he felt protective of his mother yet unable to intervene or even call the police (the phone had been disconnected). Following this instance of abuse and a particularly aggressive encounter with a teen near his home, Patrick was temporarily placed in the care of an aunt and put under house arrest.

That was not the first time Patrick and his brother had seen a man hit their mother. Her three husbands and many boyfriends had included several batterers, and the question whether any of these men had physically abused Patrick remained unclear. According to Patrick, his father left home before he was born.

Patrick's teachers referred him to an in-school program called Refocus, designed for students with disciplinary problems. And then, like many other students in his middle school, Patrick began participating in the mentoring program in sixth grade. The mentoring program coordinator, Pam Lungren, recalls that Patrick became embroiled in two or three fights each week, because he "had a really hard time interpreting the behaviors of other kids. An innocent bump in the hall would be taken as a hostile push and would quickly escalate into a fistfight. He was fighting a lot for the first month and a half of school, and he was hardly ever in class. He was suspended a week for fighting, and he was in Refocus constantly."

Most of the participants in the mentoring program had been identified by their teachers as likely to benefit from weekly, hour-long meetings with individual volunteers. Despite his fighting and suspensions, Patrick's teachers had somehow seen him having the will to improve and the capacity to thrive under a better set of circumstances. Patrick was paired with Walter Pearson, a 59-year-old economics professor at the nearby university. A married father of two grown children, Walter's tall frame and silver hair give him a distinguished presence. "My daughter mentored a girl from the age of ten until college," Walter recalled, "and her positive experiences had some influence on my decision to get involved."

Patrick seemed open to the relationship and won Walter over from the start. "We would play games and talk about life at the house and grades and stuff like that," recalls Walter. Within a few weeks the conversation turned to Patrick's fighting. Although Walter grew up on a farm in Ohio and admits to never having had a fistfight, he felt ready to tackle this problem. When Patrick confessed to him that he really did not want to fight, Walter suggested that Patrick consider telling himself, "I will not fight" every time he stepped through a doorway when entering or leaving a room. In a separate conversation, Patrick mentioned this strategy, adding, "This is a really good way to remember. Walter thought of it."

Walter also thought of wrestling as a means of channeling and controlling Patrick's physical responses. As Walter explains, "In wrestling you're going to get knocked on your butt numerous times; and you can't get mad, you just have to get up and keep working." Since Patrick was responsive to the suggestion, Walter helped pave the way. He got information, checked with coaches, arranged a stipend to cover the costs of Patrick's uniform and equipment and, as was required, obtained a copy of his birth certificate from his mother.

The wrestling strategy seemed to work magic. "I don't know whether I want to take credit for this," Walter confides, "but as the year went on the fighting gradually decreased and things got better." Patrick reported that things improved at home as well. He argued less with his brother, and his relationship with his mother improved. "I don't think I drive her *quite* as crazy these days," he said, grinning.

Except during summer break, Patrick and Walter have met weekly for a year and a half. Around Christmastime, participants in the program met at the school for a celebration, and as Patrick and Walter walked together on the way to the cafeteria, their mutual affection was apparent to observers. Patrick seemed to swell with pride when Walter put his arm on his shoulder. In the lunchroom, Walter gave Patrick his Christmas present, a Harry Potter book, and they began to talk about their relationship. Although Patrick said that he could tell that Walter cares about him from "how he looks at me," Walter stated that he likes to reinforce this message through regular e-mails. "I like to put the really positive and encouraging stuff in bright colors."

The conversation somehow shifted to what each of them would do if they had a jillion dollars. In Patrick's case, "Well, if I had a jillion dollars, I would visit my sister with Walter and show him what she is like." Walter responded, "Oh that would be cool, I'd like to do that. I was thinking that we'd go in the mountains for a week-long camping trip." Walter looked at Patrick and noted that he "usually has that big smile on his face and he's really outgoing." As Patrick continued to smile, Walter added, "and he's got that great personality."

"I'm also a wrestler," Patrick chimed in.

How Does It Work?

How is it that, after years of witnessing violence and embarking on a path toward delinquency, Patrick could be so deeply affected by this rather circumscribed relationship with a total stranger? How do such relationships between youths and caring adults actually bring about change?

Most of the research on mentoring has been driven by the concept of resilience. Researchers who work within this framework attempt to understand how youth overcome profoundly difficult life circumstances. Over the past thirty years, researchers focusing on a variety of situations, including war, natural disasters, family violence, extreme poverty, and parental mental illness have uncovered traits, conditions, and situations that enable vulnerable children and youth to achieve healthy outcomes despite these profound risks.[1] Consistently, three clusters of protective factors have been recognized as fostering psychological resilience: (1) *characteristics of the individual,* such as intelligence and an appealing disposition, (2) *characteristics of the family,* such as its consistent and close relationships and socioeconomic advantages, and (3) *characteristics of the community*, such as bonds to nonrelated adults who are positive role models, connections with community organizations, good schools.[2]

Although the influence of the first two types of factors in this triad of protective factors has been fairly well established, relatively few studies have focused specifically on the protective qualities of support outside the family.[3] For example, at the 2001 annual meetings of the Society for Research on Child Development and the American Psychological Association, the programs indexed hundreds of sessions on parents and peers but only one session at each meeting on youth mentoring. This disproportion suggests a bias in Western culture that may help explain the neglect of mentoring relationships by researchers.

In Western societies, parents are considered solely responsible for their children; the involvement of other adults is often met with suspicion and discomfort.[4] And within the scholarly literature on child development, attention to maternal influences during early childhood has dominated developmental psychology. By contrast, there is no theoretical framework to guide research questions on the influence of adults who are not parents. Nor do we have an adequate theory about the influence of adults throughout the life span, not just during early childhood.[5]

Compounding these problems for researchers is the hyperbole that often surrounds mentoring programs. Unsubstantiated claims about mentoring's effectiveness have lent a patina of superficiality to the field that discourages investigators from pursuing serious studies. And when researchers do persevere to undertake complex analyses, the "good-news-only" mentality within the media tends to undermine the impact of any legitimate empirical findings they may report.

Despite these problems, researchers working in a broad array of disciplines have consistently noted the importance of nonparent adults in the lives of youths. In his pioneering work, Norman Garmezy observed that resilient children often had at least one significant adult in their lives. As a result, he noted, "the achieving youngsters seemed to hold a more positive attitude toward adults and authority figures in general."[6] Garmezy reviewed the literature on children in war, looking at studies of how boys and girls in Europe and Israel adapted to the stress of war. In addition to parents, the studies pointed to the significance of nonfamily adults as prime factors in how children respond. "Such adults," Garmezy concluded, "provide for the children a representation of their efficacy and the demonstrable ability to exert control in the midst of upheaval. From that standpoint, the sense of confidence in the adult community provides a support system of enormous importance to the well-being of children."[7]

The psychologist Michael Rutter observed that vulnerable children with "one good relationship" were less likely to develop behavior problems than others.[8] Rutter and his colleague Henri Giller noted that minority children of low-income, divorced, or separated parents were less likely to drop out of school if positively influenced by extended family members and other caring adults. This led them to speculate about the importance of situations "where good relationships outside the family can have a protective effect similar to that which apparently stems from within the immediate family."[9]

Emmy Werner and Ruth Smith reached similar conclusions in their groundbreaking thirty-year study of children on the Hawaiian Island of Kauai.[10] Compared with their less successful peers, resilient youth sought support more often from nonparent adults. In fact, without exception, all the children who thrived had at least one nonparent adult who provided consistent emotional support. Many recent studies have confirmed the protective influence of caring, competent adults who are not parents, particularly in the lives of children and adolescents facing extraordinary challenges.[11]

The resilience framework has provided a strong foundation for policies aimed at reducing risk and promoting competence in youth. Its emphasis on positive adaptation and areas of competence is a refreshing contrast to the more typical research that focuses on shortcomings. Rather than addressing only maladjustment and remediation, this framework shifts the discourse toward preventing disorders and enhancing growth.[12]

The ultimate goal in identifying protective factors that help young people thrive in difficult environments is to understand what makes such factors effective.[13] The question is not just *what?* but *why?* In answering this second question, most research on resilience, including work on the protective role of mentors, has come up short. Previous work on mentoring has not adequately explained how mentoring promotes change and why some adolescents benefit from the support more than others do.

A successful relationship with a caring adult may, in fact, be a byproduct of healthy development rather than a cause of it. Youth who are physically attractive or intelligent, who have engaging dispositions or intense interests (all of which are protective factors in their own right, whether or not the youth has a mentor), may be primed for higher levels of involvement with adults than are peers who lack these qualities.[14] Emmy Werner and Ruth Smith observed that youth who have thrived despite adversity tend to have hobbies or other interests and a unique capacity to engage with adults through those activities.[15]

Youth who have enjoyed relatively strong relationships in the past may be better equipped to elicit the support of nonparent adults and more willing to take healthy interpersonal risks within the relationships.[16] Those with histories of maltreatment, on the other hand, may be less willing to recruit caring adults into relationships.[17] Any overtures adults themselves make toward youth are likely to be perceived and responded to quite differently depending on the young person's state of receptiveness.

More than Mentors

The youth-resilience framework has another inherent weakness, and that is a tendency to overlook the larger social context in which mentoring relationships occur. Testimonials about powerful relationships with nonfamily adults often obscure adolescents' ongoing connections with their parents, who typically remain the most important adults in their lives. The tendency among resiliency researchers to isolate and credit mentors for positive outcomes can be insulting to the parents, teachers, and other adults who care for and guide youth through the complexities and struggles of their daily lives.[18]

After all, adolescents' chances of ever even forming ties with mentors are, to a large extent, a function of the encouragement and opportunities that their parents provide. Families characterized by sensitivity to others' ideas and needs and an ability to openly express views are more likely to encourage adolescents to become involved in positive relationships outside the family.[19] Several researchers have confirmed that adolescents with more supportive parental relationships and higher levels of shared family decision-making tend to have healthy relationships outside the family and to gravitate toward natural mentors.[20]

Parents who actively cultivate connections with well-meaning adults in their neighborhoods and channel their children to community-based recreational and social programs also greatly increase the likelihood that their children will form beneficial relationships with adults beyond the nuclear family.[21]

But even the most confident parent can feel threatened by a child's close relationships with another adult. Parents who enjoy positive relationships with their children may see outside adults as unnecessary intrusions, whereas parents who are struggling to connect may feel usurped. Even when parents refrain from acting on their jealousy, hurt, or resentment, they may telegraph their feelings in ways that subtly undermine the bond with a mentor.

Enlisting one's child in programs such as Big Brothers Big Sisters takes perseverance, organization, and tolerance, not to mention a willingness to undergo the intense scrutiny of home visits and interviews. Many parents harbor fears that home visitors or mentors will be judgmental or make unfair assumptions about their family circumstances or parenting practices. One mother explained how this fear and discomfort—often unacknowledged—had kept many of her friends from signing their children up for mentoring programs. "You just never know what your kid is gonna say when he is sitting at a ball game eating a hot dog with his mentor!"

Family mobility reduces an adolescent's chances of having a long-term relationship with a nonparent adult. And neighborhood instability is another important risk factor. In urban communities plagued by crime or other dangerous conditions, many parents sequester their children in their homes, greatly reducing opportunities for contact with adults outside the home and school.[22] When families, schools, churches, and civic organizations disintegrate, teenagers often have no adults available to offer counsel as problems arise.

So to summarize, the likelihood that an adolescent will encounter a mentor is increased by a great number of individual and environmental factors. Ignoring these factors and focusing too much on the resilient characteristics of some youth can inadvertently lead to blaming adolescents for not finding mentors. A more subtle analysis of mentoring requires that we consider not only individual differences among youth but also the family, community, and cultural circumstances that lead youth to mentoring relationships and help sustain them over time.

What Mentoring Means in Adolescent Development

As adolescents endure the waves of change that wash over their minds and bodies during puberty, they inevitably undergo profound shifts in their sense of self and in their understanding of others—parents, teachers, siblings, and peers.[23] Discussing these important changes with their parents is not easy for most teens, in part because parents often feel responsible for their children's struggles and compelled to fix things as quickly as possible. Family members' physical proximity and vested interest in an adolescent can cause them to overreact, to become judgmental. Frank talk about sexuality and dating in particular are difficult under the best of circumstances, and parenting a teenager awash in hormones is not the best of circumstances.

Mentors have the advantage of standing outside these family struggles. They can provide a safe haven for teens to air sensitive issues, while still transmitting adult values, advice, and perspectives. This was captured in an e-mail that a 14-year-old adolescent boy sent to an administrator, expressing his appreciation for a mentoring program.

> When I first heard about the mentoring program I wondered about what it would be like to hang out with someone 15 or 30 years older. I mean, I was honestly trying to get away from my parents and all the adults who try to

> rule my life. I thought that he might just look down on me as a "teen" and I would get most of the blame and he would always be on my parents' side—I was SO wrong. I mean, Frank, my friend (I don't consider him a mentor anymore) has really been there for me. He went through tough times when he was growing up, and he can relate to how I feel and what I go through.

Another protégée described how her mentor is "always there whenever I want to talk. We talk on the phone for hours at a time. She calls me 'chatterbox.' I feel like I can open up and just tell her anything." By providing their point of view in a supportive, trusting context, mentors can help adolescents successfully balance autonomy with closeness in their interactions with their parents. And unlike parental advice, which adolescents are often quick to dismiss, guidance and encouragement from a nonparent adult is sometimes taken more to heart.

Unfortunately, when adults are scarce, adolescents often turn to their friends for support. Today's adolescents spend most of their time outside of school simply hanging out with friends.[24] But friends are often grappling with similar transformations, and they often lack the experience, knowledge, and intellectual sophistication to fully assist with identity-related issues. Moreover, shifting allegiances and issues of trust and betrayal in peer relationships make many adolescents unwilling to disclose problems and explore sensitive topics in any depth with their friends.[25]

Preteens and early teens, around 10 to 14 years of age, seem more responsive to adult influences than older adolescents, who gravitate to group-based programs, where adults are available on the sidelines but are not there necessarily for the purpose of forming close bonds.[26] Romantic involvements also compete increasingly for the attention and commitment of older adolescents, as do bonds with peers who are just good friends. Mentors of older youth tend to experience their relationships as less close and supportive than mentors of preteens do, and for this reason, among others, relationships with older adolescents are at higher risk for early termination.[27]

For all adolescents, however, the inevitable crises of identity that occur during these years create unique openings for nonparent adults, who can have a positive influence on teens as they try to understand the many relationships in their lives and explore their own sense of self. In doing so, nonparent adults can fill a unique niche for youths, somewhere between their parents and their peers.

What Makes Mentoring Work

Mentors appear to affect youth through some combination of support and role modeling, but relatively little attention has been paid to how these processes work to bring about positive change. This topic—the very heart of change—has been the centerpiece of my research for over a decade.

I have concluded that mentors can influence their protégés' development in three important ways (see Figure 1):

- by enhancing social skills and emotional well-being
- by improving cognitive skills through dialogue and listening
- by serving as a role model and advocate.

Mentors whose influence extends into more than one of these three arenas are likely to have the greatest impact on adolescents' development.[28] I will explore each of these topics in the sections that follow. But first, it is important to note that none of these beneficial changes can occur until the mentor and protégé establish an emotional bond.

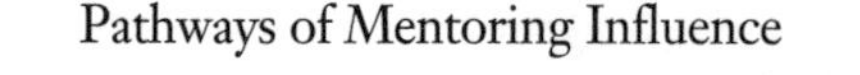

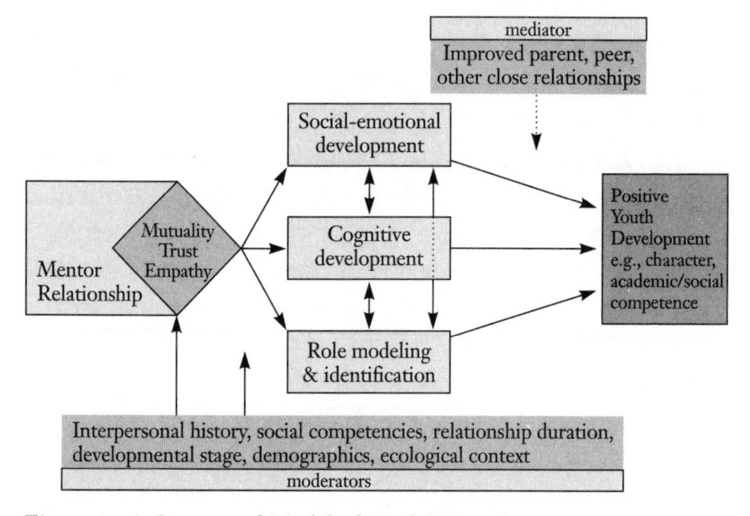

Figure 1 A Conceptual Model of Youth Mentoring

Most people would agree that a necessary condition for an effective relationship is that the two people involved feel connected—that there is mutual trust and a sense that one is understood, liked, and respected. Without some connection, the dynamics that make mentoring relationships effective are unlikely ever to occur. Adolescents often describe feeling safe in expressing their feelings and thoughts to their mentors. In this nonjudgmental, nonthreatening context they can begin to think critically about their connections to the world and their identity within it. The research literature bears them out: the "active ingredient" in a good mentoring relationship is a close, trusting connection. After examining over 600 pairs, Carla Herrera and her colleagues observed that "at the crux of the mentoring relationship is the bond that forms between the youth and mentor. If a bond does not form, then youth and mentors may disengage from the match before the mentoring relationship lasts long enough to have a positive impact on youth."[29]

Researchers who make it their business to study close relationships tend to agree that strong bonds depend on the ability to understand and respond empathetically to others' experiences.[30] Empathy has been described as "the recognition of the self in the other," or as listening with "not only eyes and ears, but also hearts and minds."[31] Judith Jordan explains that empathy requires a delicate balance between emotions and thought so as to neither lose oneself nor be overly distant and intellectual.[32] Empathy is captured well in Mitch Albom's best-selling book about his mentor, *Tuesdays with Morrie.*

> Those who sat with him [Morrie] saw his eyes go moist when they spoke about something horrible, or crinkle in delight when they told him a really bad joke. He was always ready to openly display the emotion so often missing from my baby boomer generation. We are great at small talk: "What do you do?" "Where do you live?" But really listening to someone—without trying to sell them something, pick them up, recruit them, or get some kind of status in return—how often do we get this anymore? I believe many visitors in the last few months of Morrie's life were drawn not because of the attention they wanted to pay him but because of the attention he paid to them.

As this example suggests, a mentor-protégé relationship is not necessarily mutually empathic. The protégé's life is center-stage. Nonetheless, there is often mutual caring, respect, and understanding; and in that sense, the mentor and protégé each benefit from the relationship. Additionally, a strong connection does not necessarily depend on divulging personal confidences or making sophisticated interpretations about problems.[33] And a close bond is not necessarily free of conflict. In fact, conflict and its successful resolution can help people understand and confront their differences.[34]

Bonds between mentors and protégés tend to deepen with time. Thus, another important dimension of this connection is continuity and a motivation on the part of both the protégé and mentor to remain responsive to change in the relationship. Finally, an adolescent's bond is specific to one mentor and not interchangeable with anyone else. This topic will be explored in greater depth in Chapter 3. But for now let's return to the three areas in which mentors bring about constructive change: in social and emotional development, in cognitive development, and in role modeling and advocacy.

Enhancing Social and Emotional Development

When adolescents develop close connections with mentors, their ability to connect with other adults, especially their parents, also improves. This change is often noticed by both parents and program personnel. One case manager observed, "Parents sometimes tell me that the mentoring program has done more for their relationship with their child than any amount of family counseling they had in the past." Although some adolescents who are referred to mentoring programs already have close relationships with their parents, others are more distant. Some adolescents have suffered maltreatment in their homes, but many others have simply grown apart from their parents and are inhibited and uncertain about their ability to establish new relationships, especially with adults. Through consistently warm and accepting interactions with their mentors, protégés can begin to recognize the enormous potential that exists in close relationships and to open themselves up more to the people around them.

Heinz Kohut has argued that close relationships can be therapeutic, helping people realize "that the sustaining echo of empathic resonance is indeed available in the world."[35] Consistent with this observation, Grossman and Tierney found that youth with mentors reported better relationships with both parents and peers than those in the control group, including greater feelings of trust and openness to deeper communication.[36] Melanie Styles and Kristine Morrow concluded that the experience of a trusting and consistent mentor relationship led to better outcomes among youth.[37]

This was vividly demonstrated in Patrick's case. As his relationship with Walter deepened, his defensiveness toward his peers softened. When an adolescent feels safe and accepted in the presence of a mentor, a fuller range of feelings and thoughts, and different ways of relating and being related to, can grow.

A New Model for Relationships

The perspectives of attachment theory offer another way to understand how positive relationships can change adolescents' perceptions of themselves and their relationships. According to attachment theory, children form their conceptions of relationships through their early experiences with primary caregivers, which John Bowlby called attachment figures.[38] Sensitive and responsive care-giving engenders in children a sense of self-worth: they see themselves as worthy of love, and others as trustworthy to give love and to be consistently available in times of need.

Unreliable or insensitive care-giving engenders insecurity in children. They feel anger and disappointment, and they view others in their lives as unlikely to meet their needs. These beliefs and expectations, sometimes called working models, are believed to exist on a largely unconscious level but to influence interpersonal relationships throughout and beyond childhood.[39]

Attachment issues often become salient during adolescence, when changing relationships with parents and peers evoke questions about identity and intimacy and challenge adolescents to consider others' perspectives. Not surprisingly, adolescents with deep-seated insecurities about relationships tend to be more vulnerable to self-criticism and distress. Mentors can help these adolescents create strategies for coping with stress without coming down so hard on themselves, and in certain cases mentors can serve as alternative or secondary attachment figures.[40] In doing so, they can help adolescents to realign their conceptions of themselves in relation to others.

Working models of relationships are difficult to change, but not impossible. Youth can adapt to changing life circumstances, such as connecting with a teacher or coach.[41] In fact, this stage of development may be uniquely well-suited for revision and reconceptualization of one's working models of relationships, since so much rapid change of some kind is inevitable during these years.[42]

Mentors can positively influence adolescents' relationships—even those adolescents whose ability to make attachments is already strong and who are generally able to maintain a firm sense of themselves.[43] By acting as a sounding board and providing a model for effective communication, mentors can help adolescents better understand, more clearly express, and more effectively control both their positive and their negative emotions.[44] Moreover, parental advice and suggestions become more difficult to dismiss when they are reinforced by an adolescent's mentor.

In a recent study, my colleagues and I tested some of the social and emotional effects of mentoring. We found, first, that mentoring relationships led to increases in the levels of intimacy, communication, and trust that adolescents felt toward their parents. These improvements, in turn, led to positive changes in a wide array of areas, such as the adolescents' sense of self-worth and scholastic achievement.[45]

Despite the consistency of our findings across several studies, it remains to be determined how these processes work for different youth. Mentoring relationships may lead to improvements in parental relationships simply by reducing tensions or promoting better communication or through more fundamental shifts in adolescents' perceptions of themselves and their ability to form and sustain relationships.

Improvements in adolescents' sense of self-worth could be understood as an internalization of their mentors' positive appraisals of them. The sociologist Charles Horton Cooley, writing about the "looking glass self" around the turn of the twentieth century, theorized that significant others become social mirrors into which adolescents look to form opinions of themselves. Those opinions are then integrated into the adolescents' sense of self-worth.[46] George Herbert Mead and others built on this theory, suggesting that adolescents try to imagine how they are perceived from the perspective of significant others.[47] Thus, adolescents might project themselves into the role of their mentors and appraise situations and themselves from the mentors' standpoint. In this sense, adolescents' views of themselves are partially a "reflected appraisal" of others' judgments of them.

If a mentor views a youth positively, that can start to change the youth's view of herself and can even start to change the way she thinks parents, peers, teachers, and others view her. In such cases, a mentor's positive appraisal can gradually become incorporated into the adolescent's stable sense of self. This self-appraisal process is facilitated by the growing capacity of adolescents to understand the world from the perspective of others and to view themselves from that point of view. Whatever the underlying processes, it appears that guidance and support from an adult outside the home can lead to improvements in an adolescent's sense of self in relationship.

These findings should assuage parents' fears that mentors will usurp their influence. Rather than acting as a substitute for intimacy and communication with parents, mentoring appears to produce positive effects that reverberate back, ultimately drawing adolescents and their parents closer together.

Although mentoring programs have not always involved parents and families in a comfortable or coherent manner, program personnel should remain aware of the ways that successful mentoring relationships can improve family dynamics, and they should capitalize on that possibility. Caseworkers and mentors need to acknowledge parents' emotional conflicts around enlisting their children in the program. They ought to arrange for regular feedback sessions in which the parents' perspectives and adolescents' needs and accomplishments are discussed. Some mentoring programs have gone so far as to extend case management to parents—who are often struggling with financial and emotional difficulties of their own—as a way of solidifying parents' commitment to the program. If a parent feels involved in—as opposed to shut out by—the process that brings another adult into a child's life, the parent is more likely to reinforce the mentor's positive influences. When relationships with parents are valued by all parties in the program, adolescents are less likely to feel trapped by competing loyalties.

Bowlby once remarked that humans seem "happiest and able to deploy their talents to best advantage when they are confident that, standing behind them, there are one or more trusted persons who will come to their aid should difficulties arise."[48] To the extent that mentors and parents can work together to provide this backup, adolescents are likely to show improvements in the social and emotional domains of their lives.

Improving Cognitive Skills through Meaningful Conversation

The positive social and emotional changes described above are deeply intertwined with adolescents' developing cognitive skills. Adolescence is a time of significant mental as well as emotional growth—a time when young people become both more self-reflective and more self-aware. Over the course of adolescence, youth typically experience improvements in basic cognitive processes (such as the brain's speed, efficiency, and capacity in processing information); in knowledge and thinking skills (such as abstract representations, simultaneous consideration of multiple issues, relative rather than absolute conceptions); and in the ability to evaluate one's own thoughts and feelings for consistency, gaps, and accuracy.[49]

What's more, researchers believe that this mental and emotional growth is intertwined with adolescents' views of themselves and society. In fact, they believe that social interaction—particularly ordinary conversations—plays a major role in honing and improving adolescents' mental abilities.[50] The Russian psychologist L. S. Vygotsky described a "zone of proximal development" in which learning takes place for young people. Think of the zone of proximal development as a psychological stretch: it's beyond what a young person can do when problem-solving on his or her own but within the range of what he or she can do while working under adult guidance or with more capable peers.[51] When youth are stretched by their adult or peer interactions into this zone, their own mental and emotional capacities improve and grow. What is today a stretch facilitated by interaction with others can, in the future, become part of a youth's own capability.

This research has important implications for mentoring. It suggests that adolescents' capacity for critical thinking and self-awareness can be increased through ongoing conversations on meaningful topics with their mentors. Conversations where mentors listen to, attempt to understand, and show respect for what adolescents have to say, even if the mentors do not always agree, can provide adolescents with opportunities to think more clearly and critically about the world, to stay in touch with feelings and thoughts, and to express themselves more fully. In doing so, mentors can help adolescents test their ideas and sharpen cognitive skills that they would not use on their own, or in day-to-day conversation with their peers. Adolescents can then incorporate what they have learned from these conversations into their existing base of knowledge and competence.[52]

Opportunities for authentic conversation are particularly important for adolescents, who often hide their true feelings from their parents, teachers, friends, and others out of a fear of disapproval or rejection.[53] Given the complicated transitions that other close relationships undergo in adolescence, and the openings provided by adolescents' growing capacity for understanding and reflecting, mentors are uniquely positioned to engage their protégés in the sorts of deep, reflective conversations that can advance their critical thinking and self-awareness.[54]

Researchers have noted, however, that adolescents' expanding cognitive processes are intertwined with complex new emotions and a decreasing sense of certainty about how they fit into a world of changing relationships. As Daniel Keating observed, "New and powerful emotions challenge the adolescents' emerging rationality and search for principles, but it is on those same developing cognitive skills that the adolescent must rely to make sense of unexpectedly complex feelings."[55] If mentors are to facilitate cognitive development, they must also be equipped to engage fully with the adolescents on an emotional level. In this sense, a trusting relationship provides the scaffolding onto which the adolescent can acquire and refine thinking skills.[56] Along similar lines, adolescents can use their increasing intellectual sophistication to manage their emotional experiences.[57]

Role Modeling and Advocacy

Adolescence is a time when young people begin to think about the adults they may become, and to wonder how they might fit into the adult world of work and responsibility. Role modeling, in which mentors exemplify the sorts of knowledge, skills, and behavior that adolescents hope to someday acquire, can be a powerful instrument for positive development.

Mentors can become an enormous asset for lower-income youth who may have limited contact with positive role models outside the immediate family and may believe that their opportunities for success are restricted.[58] But even among middle-income youth, adult occupations and skills can seem obscure and out of reach. Mentors can serve as concrete examples of career success, demonstrating qualities that adolescents might wish to emulate.[59] By observing and comparing their own performance to that of their mentors, adolescents can begin to adapt their behaviors and adopt new ones.

This modeling process is thought to be reinforced through mentors' emotional support and verbal feedback.[60] Freud described this as an identification process in which individuals internalize the traits, attitudes, and behaviors of those they wish to emulate.[61] Similarly, Kohut described the ways in which children and adolescents attach themselves to an idealized parental "imago" whose qualities they integrate into their own personalities.[62] Through the process of identifying with mentors, youth's early internalizations can begin to shift, bringing about changes in how they perceive themselves and their social roles.

Even when mentors do not serve as direct models, they can be influential in helping adolescents focus on a brighter future. They can advocate on behalf of their protégés, opening doors to new opportunities and helping them to establish and make use of connections in the community, such as little leagues, neighborhood associations, religious programs, and parent-teacher organizations. These sources of support, encouragement, and trust make up the "social capital" of a community, and the denser the networks, the better for young people. Social capital has been associated with school success above and beyond the contribution of family income, parents' education, or household composition. Mentors can help youth who might otherwise be adrift to make these important connections with other caring, cooperating adults within their own community.[63]

Mentors can act as an audience from whom adolescents seek attention and approval, or they can help adolescents to define an appropriate audience.[64] Mentors can help adolescents to identify and become part of more socially desirable or higher achieving peer groups (for example, students in an honors class, athletes, or musicians). Mentors can encourage their protégés to avoid peers who engage in destructive behavior, or to resist their negative influence. Researchers have found that adolescents with natural mentors are less likely to engage in problem behaviors, regardless of the behaviors of their close friends and family members.[65] As was demonstrated with Nancy and Angela, mentors can hold their protégés to higher standards or introduce new visions of what adolescents can achieve. Thus, through role modeling, social comparison and reinforcement, skill building, and shaping norms and values, mentors can be a positive force for change.

General beliefs about self-efficacy can become even more influential and motivating when they are linked to specific possibilities for the future, or "possible selves."[66] Such possibilities, which often arise as adolescents observe and compare the adults in their lives, can inform their decisions and behavior. This notion of possible selves is similar to Daniel Levinson's description of the "imagined self," which becomes refined over time and motivates adolescents as they make the transition into early adulthood.[67] A mentor in Minneapolis described how she helped her protégé begin to imagine her own future: "Sara's family was pretty fragmented and she was staying with different relatives—pretty much getting lost in the shuffle. On her fifteenth birthday, I asked her if she had thought about career paths, and she just drew a complete blank. I didn't know where to start but I thought that maybe, by visiting some work settings—hospitals, banks, libraries—and talking with me about my job [stock broker], she could learn about different days in the workplace." With help from her mentor, by the time Sara entered her senior year of high school she had plans to apply to a local business college.

This process of constructing, valuing, and believing in possible selves is intertwined with adolescents' developing thinking skills. With their increased perspective-taking abilities, adolescents become actively involved in shaping and evaluating the course of their lives. Because adolescents also try to imagine how others view them, they may try to evaluate their possible future roles and life courses from the perspective of their mentors.[68]

Of course, these role modeling, shaping, and planning processes are not without tensions and difficulties, particularly when they lead adolescents down paths that are different from those of family members. Such differences may make it more difficult to establish trust and may diminish the extent to which adolescents can identify with their mentors. In some instances, minority, lower-income, or immigrant adolescents may feel tensions between their mentors' vision of success and their family's values, particularly if their mentors are middle-class and white.[69]

Elizabeth DeBold and colleagues have described this situation as a "dilemma of connection," or a forced choice between competing loyalties.[70] Susan Harter has argued that when an individual's self-concept is linked to the reactions of significant others, some adolescents might create a "false self" which is not grounded in their actual experiences. Mentors should remain sensitive to these dilemmas and calibrate the pace and direction of their influence accordingly.[71]

Additional Considerations

The emotional, social, cognitive, and role-modeling processes I have described in this chapter work in concert with one another over time. An adolescent's selection of a mentor as a role model or source of emotional support often coincides with a growing ability to make comparisons across relationships and to recognize parental imperfections—an outgrowth of the youth's increased capacity for logical and abstract reasoning.

Adolescents who have enjoyed good relationships with their parents may be drawn to adults as role models and confidants. The relationship with a mentor may center more on the acquisition of skills and the advancement of critical thinking than on emotional problems. Those who have experienced unsatisfactory parental ties may develop more intense bonds with their mentors, which satisfy their social and emotional needs. Immigrant youths, many of whom have suffered long separations from their parents, may gravitate to mentors for compensatory emotional support. Mentors can provide these adolescents with a safe haven for learning new cultural norms and practices, as well as with information that is vital to success in schools.[72]

Because older adolescents tend to be less interested in establishing intimate emotional ties with nonparental adults, they may choose to focus instead on the vocational skill-building and role-modeling aspects of a mentoring relationship.[73] In addition to different reactions depending on age, adolescents react differently depending on their gender. Many adolescents who are referred to mentoring programs are living in single-parent homes headed by the mother; this is the situation of a majority of youth in Big Brothers Big Sisters programs. A mother might refer her son to a program in response to what she perceives as a need for a male role model. This may be particularly true as the son reaches early adolescence and his peers become more influential. Alternatively, a mother might refer her daughter to a female mentor, in response to difficulties in their mother-daughter relationship. My colleagues and I found that adolescent girls who were referred to Big Brothers Big Sisters programs had lower levels of communication, trust, and intimacy with their mothers than did adolescent boys.[74] For young women and others who are struggling to connect with their parents, the mentor relationship may be defined less by any particular activity or skill than by interpersonal needs.

The many influences in mentoring raise important questions about how to define success and measure results. Researchers often conceive of mentoring relationships in narrow terms, such as an influence on specific behaviors or symptoms. As the above discussion implies, however, changes in youth vary tremendously; they are sometimes complex and subtle, and they may emerge over a relatively long period of time. Although different youths have different needs, all youth in mentoring programs will ultimately benefit if researchers and practitioners can gain a deeper understanding of the processes that govern mentoring relationships.

Benefits to the Mentor

The quotation from *Charlotte's Web* at the beginning of this chapter raises, and then helps us answer, the question, "What's in it for mentors?" The basic premise that an emotional connection lies at the heart of this kind of intervention underscores its reciprocal nature. Yet the emotional rewards that mentors receive are rarely considered in writings on mentoring. Instead, the process tends to be conveyed in terms of the adult selflessly giving to the protégé in a one-sided relationship. It would be a mistake, however, to assume that the mentor gets relatively little from the relationship. And indeed, when one member derives little or no benefit from a relationship, it will become unstable and may disintegrate.[75] One-sided relationships drain mentors of enthusiasm and leave protégés feeling burdened by the imbalance. On the other hand, when adolescents see that admired adults find it personally rewarding to spend time with them, they feel a new surge of self-worth and empowerment.

Frank Riessman's helper-therapy principle—that people help themselves through the process of being genuinely helpful to others—is particularly applicable to understanding the considerable rewards of mentoring.[76] The sense of efficacy and pride that can come from being admired and helpful may well be a driving force in the positive changes commonly observed in mentors' lives.[77] In a recent *Newsweek* editorial, Jane

Armstrong described the joy she felt after arranging an informational visit with a pediatrician for her protégé, Risa, and then witnessing Risa's unbridled enthusiasm for a possible career in medicine. "I looked over at Risa's beautiful face. I wanted to hit the brakes, pull the car over, stare at her and expand time because I knew nothing before or since in my shaky career as a mentor would ever come close to this moment. Risa's world had just opened up, had become huge and complicated and full of possibilities, and I was there to see it happen."[78]

A similar experience is detailed in Jon Katz's book *Geeks*, in which he chronicles the ascension of two somewhat adrift youth into computer jobs and college careers. Through the process of writing the book, Katz's relationship with one of the boys, Jesse, deepened into a close bond. As Katz describes: "When we first met, I could see that he expected me to vanish at any moment. Over time he came—cautiously—to see that I wouldn't. His trust in me was touching, my faith in him absolute . . . His passion to move forward with his life overcame even his fearsome pride . . . and he has repaid me in many ways."[79]

Although none of Jesse's relatives or friends had gone to college, and his family had been torn apart by difficulties, Katz encouraged him to pursue an education and shepherded him through the University of Chicago's application process. In this passage, Katz describes his reaction on receiving a voice mail from Jesse:

> I played it back. It was Jesse, speaking in a voice tinged with a kind of excitement I'd never heard before, that he'd never permitted himself. He was breathless, childlike, speaking twice as fast as normal—"Hey Jon, this is Jesse. I just got a letter from the University of Chicago to-

day, and it's a letter of acceptance. I got the fat envelope! You give me a call when you get in. Bye." My first reaction was disbelief, followed by rich, inexpressible joy. I called Jesse up and we screamed "Awesome!" and "Cool!" at one another for five solid minutes. Then I had to get off the phone or I would have gotten squishy . . . I played the message several times, sending Jesse's words rolling down the meadow, across the valley, out into the world, even though there was nobody within miles who'd hear it. I was glad he wasn't there. He disliked any show of emotion, and I would have had to feign restraint. Instead my eyes welled up. For Jesse, and, a bit, for me.

In addition to the sheer joy, pride, and inspiration that sometimes accompany mentoring, many volunteers benefit from the social interaction. Other rewards can include improved health, self-esteem, insight into one's own childhood or children, and public recognition. Erik Erikson has described the importance of "generativity"—giving loving care to others and making societal contributions—as necessary for healthy development in later life.[80] Through mentoring, adults can blend their past experiences and wisdom. This can be true particularly for older adults, for whom the experience can provide a sense of accomplishment and offset feelings of stagnation and loss.[81] Research has shown that older adults who volunteer feel greater satisfaction with their lives and enjoy improved health.[82]

Susan Weinberger, who recently completed a survey at Allstate Insurance company, found that 75 percent of employees who became mentors to elementary school children reported that the activity improved their attitude at work.[83] More generally, volunteering can have the effect of creating a common fabric in communities—a breaking down of the artificial we-them distinctions between more and less privileged members of society.

Recognition of the mutual benefits of volunteering is at the very heart of the concept of learning through public service—a combination of academic lessons with community involvement that has become extremely popular on college campuses during the last decade, and a graduation requirement in many high schools. For example, many high schools in Massachusetts require 40 hours of public service to graduate. This approach has been widely advocated by both scholars and college administrators as a way to enhance students' academic engagement, performance, and knowledge of the outside world while increasing their appreciation of the responsibilities of living in a democracy.[84] In the following chapters, I will describe some of these mutual benefits as well as some of the costs that arise in mentoring.

3

The Risks of Relationships

Make a habit of two things—to help, or at least to do no harm.

Hippocrates

Thirteen-year-old Cameron Nichols was the envy of his neighborhood when his mentor, Rick, picked him up at his home for their first outing. Cameron had already bragged to his younger brother and neighbors that his mentor was a firefighter, but when Rick pulled up to his apartment building in a fire truck, Cameron was floored. He beamed as he waved goodbye to the small crowd of neighbors who had gathered on the sidewalk. But behind his exuberant smile, Lillian Nichols sensed her son's anxiety. As the truck turned the corner on that warm autumn day, Lillian's eyes filled with tears. "Lord," she prayed to herself, "please let this work out for Cameron."

Cameron needed a break as far as relationships were concerned. Although it had been nine years since his biological father, a police officer, had moved out, Cameron still felt the sting of loss. "Cameron was very close to Ed [his father] and, in some ways, still is. He would do just about anything to get Ed's attention, and was so happy when they were together . . . But Ed was an alcoholic, so temper and mood swings always clouded his moments of kindness. I couldn't deal with it anymore . . . but try explaining this to a first grade boy."

Visitation was arranged, and every other weekend Cameron stayed with his paternal grandmother and saw his father. After only a few months, however, his father was often late or absent from the visit. Weekends began to come and go with no trace of Ed. Sometimes Cameron would not hear from his father for two to three months at a time. According to his mother, Cameron's painful weekends of waiting and anticipation seemed to drain him of energy for school or friendships. He put up intense struggles each morning, and his teachers reported that he seemed to suffer through days in a state of loneliness and distraction.

Desperate to help her son, Lillian sought out a mentoring program at Cameron's middle school. Cameron was assigned to Rick, a kind and respectable man who took an immediate interest in the boy. "Cameron was definitely a happier child when he was meeting with Rick," recalls Lillian, "and he didn't complain about going to school. On the days he saw Rick he'd be really excited."

Rick seemed to relish the mentoring role as well, taking Cameron to the fire station and high school baseball games, throwing passes with him, and making plans for summer outings. But by late spring, after nearly seven months of consistently meeting for an hour or more each week, difficulties began to overwhelm Rick. His wife's mother developed a serious illness, and he was given additional responsibilities at work. His relationship with Cameron was one of the first casualties of these new stresses.

"I wasn't aware that Rick wasn't showing up, at least not at first," said Lillian. "I would ask Cameron if he had seen Rick and he wouldn't respond. His not wanting to tell me is the same thing with his dad. Sometimes his dad will see him and sometimes he just doesn't bother. But Cameron is always willing to make excuses for him. I see that same protecting with Rick."

As the calls became less frequent, Cameron began to show more serious signs of distress. Lillian recalls, "There were problems in school. I was getting reports from his teachers that he would spend a whole lot of time staring out the window. And he wouldn't study at home either; he was just glued to the window. He has become more irritable, more inward. He shuts himself in his bedroom and hates to go to school."

When the coordinator of the mentoring program tried to intervene, Rick promised to be more consistent and resisted her suggestions to formally terminate the relationship. But he could no longer sustain steady contact. Ignoring the signs, Cameron continued to hold out hope. As the school year ended, he began to anticipate his summer plans. "Rick had made all sorts of promises to Cameron," reported Lillian, "water-skiing, cookouts, going fishing on some lake—then he didn't show up or call or anything . . . The low point, I think, was his thirteenth birthday. Rick called Cameron and asked him what he wanted. He said that he would come to his party. Cameron delayed the party waiting for Rick, who never did show up . . . Cameron was crushed. I think that he began to expect less of Rick after that . . . I asked him yesterday if he had seen Rick and he said no. Then, I asked, 'Did you see him last week?' and he said, 'I don't think so.'"

Hoping to ease her son's pain, Lillian began to explore the possibility of finding another mentor for Cameron on her own. She even approached the youth leader at her church, who agreed to give it a try. But when she brought it up, Cameron insisted, "No, I really like Rick." In tears, Lillian responded, "Cameron, this is not your fault. This is hard on any kid and I don't want you putting any more of this on yourself."

Disruptive Ties

Painful as it was, Cameron's situation is far from unique. Whereas some pairs meet regularly for years, many mentoring relationships end much sooner. Half of all volunteer relationships dissolve within only a few months, according to some estimates.[1]

This happens for a wide variety of reasons, many of which are not the mentor's responsibility. For example, many youth in mentoring programs are from single-parent families, which tend to move around more than average.[2] Graduations, illnesses, or parental remarriages also influence adolescents' eligibility or present impediments to meetings on a regular basis.[3] In some instances, adolescents may terminate relationships in response to what they perceive as unsupportive or judgmental mentors.[4] Relationships may also fade in competition with youths' budding romances or friendships or time-consuming activities such as sports. Sometimes the adolescent's family or friends might apply pressure on the adolescent to quit the mentoring program because they feel threatened by the changes they see.

On the other hand, volunteers quit because of fear of failure or because of a perceived lack of effort or appreciation on the part of their protégés. Indeed, many adolescents enter mentoring programs with histories of inconsistent and difficult relationships, and their initial suspicions come across as indifference, defiance, and resistance. Faced with competing demands for their time, many mentors are hard pressed to persevere when the initial rewards are so low. Or they may find that the personal investment required to work with troubled adolescents exceeds their expectations, particularly if involvement is drawing them away from work and family obligations.[5] Still other mentors enter programs with unrealistic expectations, including heroic fantasies of rescuing a child from dire straits. The difficult home situation or emotional neediness of protégés may ignite painful memories in mentors or overwhelm their capacity for intimacy, causing them to withdraw from the relationship. Finally, some relationships may simply lack a basic chemistry and eventually give way to other demands.

Social exchange theorists, who believe that the survival or demise of all relationships depends largely on rewards outweighing costs, predict this instability.[6] Different rewards are essential at different stages in relationships. Volunteers and youth can be drawn to the relationship in anticipation of imagined rewards, but real rewards are needed to develop and sustain it. The positive dividends may increase as pairs move toward greater intimacy and stability. As is often the case in mentoring, however, a lack of rewards may send individuals drifting apart.

Nonetheless, because a personal relationship is at the heart of mentoring, inconsistencies and terminations can touch on vulnerabilities in youth in ways that other, less personal youth programs do not. Like Cameron, many adolescents come from single-parent homes (an eligibility requirement for some programs) and may have already sustained the loss of regular contact with their noncustodial parent, often the father. Such youth may feel particularly vulnerable to, and responsible for, problems in subsequent adult relationships.[7] Youth who have experienced unsatisfactory or rejecting parental relationships in the past may harbor fears and doubts about whether others will accept and support them.[8] When adolescents sense that their mentoring relationships are not going well—however minimal or ambiguous the signs—they may readily perceive intentional rejection.[9]

Regardless of prior histories, all youth show certain vulnerabilities to early terminations. Relative to younger children, adolescents tend to experience a greater number of negative stressors.[10] These events are often linked in some way to the normal transitions in their lives. For example, the transition to middle school might precipitate the loss of a close friendship. When terminations with mentors occur suddenly or coincide with other difficult changes, adolescents can experience significant emotional distress.

More generally, adolescence is a life stage during which issues of acceptance and rejection are paramount.[11] Feelings of belonging are central to adolescents' sense of self, which is often defined through others' eyes. Gil Noam (1997) describes adolescent identity as revolving around interpersonal issues; he humorously refers to a "wego" instead of an "ego," and observes that the central questions of early adolescence are often less "Who am I" or "What am I committed to?" and more "Where do I belong?" "What am I part of?" "Who accepts me?" "Who likes me?"[12]

Adolescents' dependence on the assessments of others can be enormously beneficial when mentoring relationships are enduring and supportive. Kind and accepting mentors can provide the nurturance, approval, and support that are incorporated into adolescents' positive self-images. But there are also risks. Mentors who are unresponsive, or who neglect or prematurely terminate relationships, can cause their protégés to perceive and incorporate disapproving or rejecting opinions into their sense of self. This, in turn, can lead to feelings of inadequacy and give rise to fears that they are unworthy of support.[13]

If adolescents have identified with their mentors and have begun to value the relationship, they are apt to feel profound disappointment if the relationship does not progress. Feelings of rejection and disappointment, in turn, can lead to a host of negative emotional, behavioral, and academic outcomes.[14]

The Duration of Relationships Matters

In an analysis of data from the national Big Brothers Big Sisters study, Jean Grossman and I looked at whether the effects of mentor relationships varied as a function of their duration. Mentored youth were categorized into four groups, depending on how long their matches had lasted: less than six months (19 percent), six to just under twelve months (36 percent), and twelve months or more (45 percent). Figure 2 depicts how treatment youth in these various groups fared in comparison with youth who did not have mentors. Youth who were in matches that terminated within the first three months suffered significantly larger drops in feelings of self-worth and perceived scholastic competence than control youth. On the other hand, youth who were in matches that lasted more than twelve months reported significantly higher levels of self-worth, social acceptance, and scholastic competence; they also reported that their relationship with their parents had improved, that school had become more rewarding, and that both their drug and alcohol use had declined.

This pattern of findings suggests that short-lived matches can have a detrimental effect on youth and that the impact of mentoring grows as the relationship matures. The same pattern of findings might have emerged, however, if youth who were particularly well adjusted were most able to sustain mentor relationships, while the less well-adjusted youth were most likely to drift away from their mentors. Even after statistically controlling for this potential selection bias, a similar pattern of findings emerged. In particular, two results stand out: shorter-lasting relationships were associated with heightened

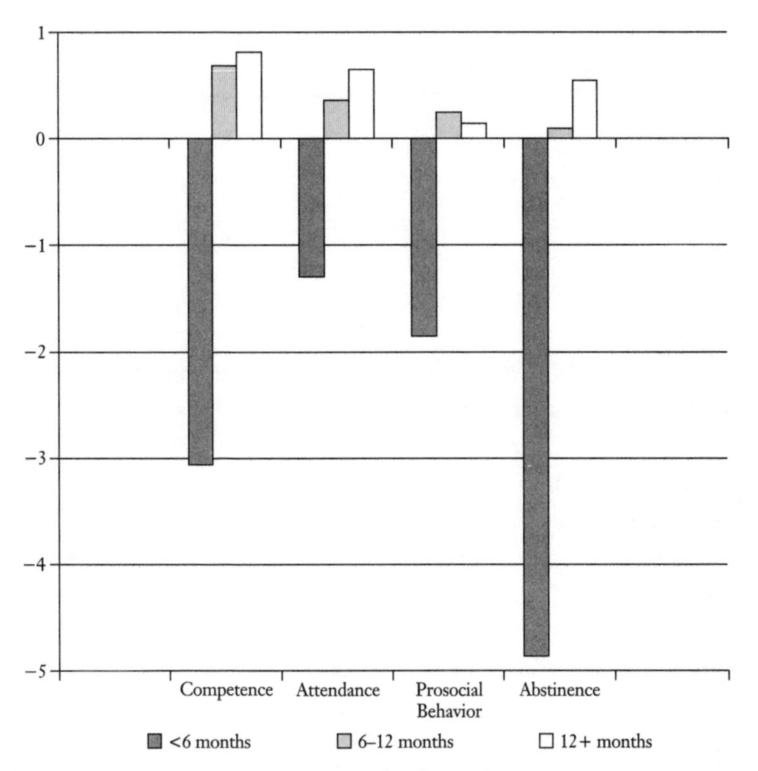

Figure 2 Outcomes as a Function of Relationship Duration

problems, and the positive effects of longer mentoring relationships increased with time.

The findings that emerged in our study seem to suggest that Cameron's situation may be playing itself out in countless subtle and not-so-subtle versions across programs. They are reminiscent of the well-known Cambridge-Somerville Youth Study, which included more than 500 at-risk boys who were randomly assigned to either a treatment or a no-treatment control condition. In the treatment condition, paid mentors were trained to meet with the boys an average of two times per month to provide tutoring, outings, and emotional support. The program lasted approximately five years (1939–1944), but the participants were traced thirty years after its termination.

The results indicated no difference between treatment and control groups in terms of criminal records, either in 1942 or in 1975–76.[15] The latter follow-up, however, did show significantly higher levels of alcoholism and mental health problems among the treatment group. Reflecting on these findings, Lawrence Sherman speculated that "the abrupt departure of these long-term counselors from the boys' lives was as damaging emotionally to the boys as a divorce or other loss of parental involvement, compounded in many cases by the boys' previous loss of their own natural fathers' support." Sherman notes that the findings could also be accounted for by selection issues—the treatment youth may have been more comfortable obtaining services.[16] It may also be the case that any positive effects in the treatment group were overshadowed by negative findings. More recent evaluations of mentoring programs hint at this possibility. In particular, Ellen Slicker and Douglas Palmer found that students who were "effectively mentored" (as measured by the quality and length of the relationship) had better academic outcomes than controls, whereas those whose relationships terminated prematurely experienced a significant decline in self-concept when compared with the students who were not mentored at all.[17]

Additional Considerations

It is also important to note that this vulnerability to negative outcomes in short-term relationships may not apply to all matches or mentoring programs. For example, some mentoring programs coincide with school calendars and have tightly stipulated endpoints of nine months or shorter that mentors and youth can anticipate from the start. Indeed, only about half of the 700 mentoring programs that were surveyed by Public/Private Ventures involved a commitment on the part of the volunteers for a year or more.[18] Since students enter short-term programs with different expectations, they are less likely to be troubled when relationships end within a year.

Similarly, more group-oriented approaches may diffuse the intensity of the mentor-protégé bond. Adolescents are often able to accept separation with relative ease—after all, most move seamlessly from one primary, and sometimes cherished, classroom teacher to the next each year. To the extent that healthy changes have been internalized and protégés do not hold themselves responsible for the terminations, they often cope quite effectively with this and subsequent losses.

And of course the end of a relationship does not necessarily imply an end to its meaning or influence. As Daniel Levinson pointed out in his study of young men's development, terminations are a natural part of mentoring relationships. In fact, following a termination, the protégé may take "the admired qualities of the mentor more fully into himself. He may become better able to learn from himself, to listen to the voices from within. His personality is enriched as he makes the mentor a more intrinsic part of himself."[19]

Finally, not all adolescents are passive victims of early terminations. Just because a negative behavior is correlated with an early termination does not necessarily mean that the termination caused the behavior. Some youth, by virtue of their emotional or behavioral profile, are ill-equipped to hold up their end of the bargain, and premature terminations may be more a symptom than a cause of their difficulties. Nonetheless, the pattern of findings presented above should give serious pause to those who would emphasize quantity over quality in mentoring programs and should encourage directors to seek ways to develop longer-lasting relationships between mentors and protégés.

Fostering Sustained Relationships

When the tool of change is a close relationship, everyone involved should proceed with care. Unfortunately, not all programs subscribe to this perspective. Indeed, moving youth off long wait lists can sometimes take priority over creating high-quality matches with a good chance of enduring. Even among the growing number of programs with careful recruitment, screening, and matching, a relatively smaller proportion devote themselves to in-depth training of volunteers. Among 700 nationally representative mentoring programs, fewer than half provided volunteers with two or more hours of training, and a distressing 22 percent offered no training whatsoever.[20] A follow-up study with this sample revealed that those mentors who attended fewer than two hours of pre-match orientation or training reported the lowest levels of satisfaction with their matches, whereas those attending six or more hours of training reported having the strongest relationships.[21]

After the initial orientation and training, levels of support to mentors tend to diminish even further. For example, in their survey of programs, Cynthia Sipe and Anne Roder found that the median ratio of mentors to paid staff was 20:1 and that only one-third of these programs contacted mentors more than once a month.[22] According to another survey by the same group, 20 percent of volunteers "almost never" talk to staff people in the programs they work with, and 9 percent have no contact with staff at all.[23] In a recent meta-analysis of over fifty mentoring programs revealed, fewer than 25 percent provided ongoing training for mentors once relationships had been established; yet the effectiveness of mentoring programs was determined in large part by the level of their commitment to the longevity of relationships.[24] The features that promote longevity in relationships have been identified by researchers, as we will see below, but they are often neglected in mentoring programs.

Cost, combined with a general reluctance to make excessive demands on volunteers, is the primary obstacle to providing more sustained involvement and infrastructure beyond the initial match.[25] In small organizations, a handful of staff members run the entire show. And in agencies of all sizes, the pressing needs to keep programs financially afloat often overshadow the more subtle demands of clients and volunteers. Since most staff work under the assumption that mentoring programs are inherently beneficial to youth, they put their limited resources into creating these new matches, rather than sustaining matches that have already been made. Funding agencies reinforce this tendency, often using the number of new matches, as opposed to their sustainability, as the measure of a program's success.

This casual attitude toward follow-up goes beyond the problem of limited resources, however. It also stems from a collective underestimation of risks. The only real danger associated with placing children in the care of unrelated adults, in the thinking of many agencies, is child molestation—a very troubling but infrequent occurrence. The disappointment and suffering of youths like Cameron goes unnoticed. These boys and girls fade quietly from programs, and the failed relationships they represent are overshadowed by the more compelling success stories of their peers. Since youth typically blame themselves when relationships fail (as do their exasperated parents in many cases), the shortcomings of programs and the volunteers they recruit are largely unnoticed. The tendency in our culture to blame the victim leads us to assume that problems in a relationship rest within the child. Faced with a challenging adolescent, adults feel justified in passing the torch to a new volunteer rather than working to repair the damaged relationship.

The result is a "place holder" mentality within programs. For example, one website advised that, "if handled well, and if a new mentor is on the scene quickly, [termination of the relationship with a mentor] can be a growth experience for the mentee." Applied to an adolescent who is grieving a lost grandparent or close friend, this attitude that relationships are virtually interchangeable can be damaging. As John Bowlby observed, "To complain because a child does not welcome being comforted by a kind but strange woman is as foolish as to complain that a young man deeply in love is not enthusiastic about some other good-looking girls."[26] In the interest of "closure," the place-holder mentality trivializes the very relationship that is at the center of change in mentoring programs. Quickly finding another skilled mentor may be the right thing to do in many cases, but the loss of the original mentor should not be brushed under the rug and forgotten.

Mentoring programs sometimes attract volunteers who turn out to be unwilling or unable to make the necessary long-term commitment. A large part of the fault lies with the programs themselves, which present mentoring to potential volunteers as a series of activities within the context of a largely symbolic relationship. Programs rarely emphasize the potential vulnerabilities of youth in their recruitment campaigns. If a mentor who does not work out can be rapidly replaced with little harm to the adolescent, the volunteer sees no real danger in giving mentoring match a try. Mentoring becomes, for many people, one of an array of volunteer activities that they find to be both personally and socially reinforcing, while carrying little risk of long-term discomfort and sacrifice.

The stakes would be raised, however, if agencies described mentoring to their potential volunteers as a connection in which the risks and improvements to youth are proportional to the length and consistency of the bond. If mentors were told that the road to establishing this connection could be a tough one—that the adolescent might very well spend the first six months testing them before offering even a shred of appreciation or authentic disclosure—many people would probably examine their motivations and commitment more carefully before volunteering.

Although not a winning marketing strategy, this description would be accurate, according to research and the experience of many people in the field. After all, why should mentoring relationships adhere to a different set of rules than other significant relationships? We do not assume that grandparents, aunts, or close friends are interchangeable; yet we sometimes make this assumption with mentors. Similarly, we all know that meaningful, close relationships—particularly with teenagers—are hard work for anyone; yet this knowledge is somehow suspended when we think of mentoring relationships.

Cultural Attitudes

This cavalier approach to mentoring reflects to some degree a general suspicion within American culture toward dependence and close relationships outside the boundaries of the immediate family. The emphasis that many practitioners and theorists of child development place on a child's early relationship with the mother renders other ties relatively trivial by comparison. This deference to family bonds is sustained by traditional neo-

Freudian psychotherapy, in which clients' feelings toward their therapists are considered to be merely diagnostic of parental relationships. The therapist remains a neutral, detached presence, and the tie between this particular therapist and this particular client is minimized.

More recent trends that approach therapy as a twelve-step process—the sort of thing that clients could learn as well from reading a how-to manual or from visiting a website as from talking with a therapist face to face—also devalue the therapeutic bond. Such "manualized" approaches are rapidly becoming the standard for psychotherapy and a mainstay of training for clinical psychologists and counselors, despite evidence that they short-circuit therapists' spontaneity, empathy, and judgment.[27] This trend is linked to a greater emphasis on cost efficiency under managed care, which has severely constrained the number of therapy sessions covered by insurance. Finally, the growing tendency to construe emotional difficulties as stemming largely from disturbed brain chemistry or genetic defects (and consequently as being most responsive to pharmaceutical treatment than to talk) further trivializes the therapist's role in healing.[28]

These trends seem to ignore the research literature, which has established significant links between the quality of therapeutic relationships and positive outcomes for clients. Indeed, in their recent review of studies that track various psychotherapeutic approaches, Alexandra Bachelor and Adam Horvath argued that a good relationship between two people is "ubiquitous and universal in all successful helping endeavors."[29] Trends in psychotherapy that valorize independence as evidence of growth while minimizing the bond between the therapist and client can lead adolescents to view adult guidance and emotional support disparagingly and lead to premature separation from the adults in their lives.[30]

Of course, these recent trends in psychotherapy merely reflect larger currents of Western thought that denigrate close relationships and community and view autonomy as the hallmark of emotional maturity. In his influential essay *On Narcissism*, Freud disparaged human dependency that extends beyond infancy. From this perspective, a mature personality and a moral character evolve only through the process of separating from others. Influential theorists such as John Bowlby, Erik Erikson, and Lawrence Kohlberg built on this framework to support a view of healthy psychological development as progressing from dependence to increasing autonomy.[31]

This perspective continues to dominate, but competing conceptual frameworks have emerged in which relations with others are considered essential to healthy development.[32] Feminist theorists have emphasized the centrality of relationships to psychological development.[33] Others have stressed that experiences in relationships throughout the life span, not just in early childhood, have an important influence on continued psychological growth.

Harry Stack Sullivan, for example, delineated a series of developmental stages that he defined in terms of changing relational needs. The transition to adolescence in particular often involves a growing closeness to individuals outside the family, including intense friendships with peers and adult role models. The failure to satisfy these needs for relationship during any one of Sullivan's stages causes loneliness, which he considered the most excruciating human experience. From Sullivan's perspective, our central need is relatedness, and the fact that we seek out closeness, despite fears of disconnection and hurt, "automatically means that loneliness is more terrible than anxiety."[34]

As Sullivan's theory suggests, the need for relationships with others is so central to development that adolescents like

Cameron are willing to expose themselves to vulnerability and anxiety in order to escape feeling alone.[35] But each subsequent disappointment only raises the level of fear and anxiety that has to be overcome in order for a person to take interpersonal risks.[36] Thus, even if a kind and reliable mentor were to walk into his life after Rick walked out, it is doubtful that Cameron would easily trust his intentions and fully engage in the relationship. Rick's inconsistencies not only caused harm in their own right; they may have foreclosed the chance for a connection that once existed in that eager 13-year-old boy.

This is not to say that Cameron will never form such a bond, but it may not occur during this critical stage of his life. Or he may enter the next relationship with a far more cautious, self-protective attitude.[37] To understand the subtle implications of this shift, let's try to imagine how Cameron felt after his mentor broke his promise to come to his thirteenth birthday party. He probably experienced a confusing combination of emotions—abandoned, humiliated, and angry with his mentor for raising his hopes and lying to him. He may have also worried that something wrong with *him* made him deserve the neglect and pain his father and mentor caused. Cameron might have felt alone in his despair and isolated from the people that he most needed. Jean Baker Miller has argued that "the most terrifying and destructive feeling that a person can experience is isolation." This is not the same as simply being alone; it is the feeling of being shut out of relationships with others. The person often feels responsible for the loneliness, yet unable to change the situation. Miller suggests that people will do almost anything to escape this combination of isolation and powerlessness.[38]

Since Cameron has little hope of changing Rick, he is likely to do his best to connect on his mentor's terms—by swallowing his anger and disappointment. His father's and his mentor's hapless behavior will not change, so he must chose to act like someone who doesn't have feelings of intense closeness, neediness, anger, hurt, or disappointment. Miller would argue that Cameron has been changed by this failed relationship into a person who can no longer relate to a caring adult in a way that would help him benefit from a mentoring program.[39]

Implications

The regular meetings between volunteer mentors and protégés eventually come to an end. In many cases, the program provides a clearly stipulated endpoint, and the mentor and the protégé are able to anticipate and frame it in ways that minimize feelings of rejection and provide a sense of closure. In some cases, informal connections may continue for decades beyond the official termination, whereas for others a complete termination is a natural step that is reached by mutual agreement.

For those who have suffered multiple separations and are unprepared for the loss, the termination can be extremely upsetting. The best way to ensure that a relationship will run its natural course is to carefully screen, train, and support both the adolescent and the mentor in the relationship, and strides have been made in this regard. Because it is impossible for program staff to predetermine the course of relationships, sensitivity to the potential vulnerabilities of adolescents to loss must be incorporated into the training of volunteers and the ongoing support that program staff offer in managing and eventually terminating relationships. In the following chapter, I will discuss some of these training issues.

4

Going the Distance

Volunteers are like gemstones. When placed in the right setting and cared for, they will shine.

—Marianne Bourgault, Volunteer Coordinator
Worcester Public Library

Carrying a large stack of folders, program director Wendy Dunn makes her way to a weekly staff meeting in the offices of her Big Brothers Big Sisters agency. She is joined in a conference room by two caseworkers, where they begin making decisions about potential mentors, youth, and matches. "The best part of my job is conceiving the matches," Wendy reflects. "It's where everything—the facts, my experience, and my intuition—all come together."

Wendy's other responsibilities—mentor recruitment, intake, screening, and training—although vitally important, seem somewhat routine by comparison. Recruitment typically occurs through public service announcements, commercials, and, most commonly, word-of-mouth.[1] Churches, business corporations, government agencies, and college campuses are deep reservoirs of potential volunteers. Of those who make an initial inquiry, only about half go on to complete an application.[2] Applicants are screened through some combination of written applications, personal interviews, reference checks, and criminal record inquiries. About 75 percent of mentoring programs use at least three of these screening techniques. Most programs provide their volunteers with some form of orientation and training, the quality and intensity of which varies widely from program to program.[3]

Youth are brought into community-based and school-based mentoring programs through a parallel process of screening, typically involving interviews with both parents and adolescents, along with questionnaires that delve into their background characteristics and the reasons for approaching the program. Since typically more women than men volunteer to be mentors, the wait list for girls is usually shorter than that for boys.[4] Within a year, however, most boys and girls get matched with mentors, and they are served in roughly equal numbers.

Many programs focus solely on mentoring, while others include mentoring as one of several components in a multifaceted approach toward helping youth navigate adolescence. Some programs pursue the general goal of promoting positive development among their clients, while others focus on education or employment. Mentoring programs vary along additional dimensions, such as adult-to-child ratio, age and gender configuration, and meeting structure.

In a typical Big Brothers Big Sisters agency, youth with severe emotional disturbances are referred to more intensive treatment interventions. As Wendy explains, "Our volunteers have big hearts, not necessarily training in child psychology or crisis management." Although such referrals are wise, some evidence suggests that youth who are at slightly elevated risk (marginally less successful academically and with somewhat lower levels of family support than their peers) are most likely to benefit from mentoring.[5] Program staff have noticed that youth who are vulnerable but have not yet succumbed to relatively severe behavioral or psychological problems often derive the greatest benefits from having a mentor. Steve Menchini, former Executive Director of Mentoring USA, described them as "the kids who have veered slightly off the sidewalk."[6] Furthermore, extracurricular activities and supportive relationships with adults tend to be more beneficial to adolescents raised in urban poverty than to lower-risk youth who are more likely to encounter supportive adults in their everyday life.[7]

The matching process at Wendy's agency involves several steps. First, caseworkers present profiles of recently approved volunteers. Then they brainstorm about particular youth who might work well with those particular adults. They read over data bases culled from questionnaires and interviews with volunteers, parents, and youth, looking for preferences that might help to narrow the pool of choices. Although most matches start with gender and geographical proximity, the preferences of parents or youth regarding race, religion, age, and interests such as sports or music often narrow the choices even further. Similarly, mentors sometimes express preferences for adolescents with particular demographic or personality characteristics.

Next, the discussion turns to how a potential protégé's family situation, life challenges, maturity, activity level, interests, and interpersonal style might mesh with those of a particular volunteer. For example, a teenage boy from the inner city who lives to play soccer but rarely speaks to adults in complete sentences might not hit it off with a polysyllabic corporate lawyer from downtown. But he just might.

Mostly, explains Wendy, it's "plain instinct. You have your intuitions about people and how they might click. I think about the kids, and whatever chords they may have struck in me about who they are or where they seemed to be. At some point in all of this, I am doing many things at once—I am remembering a lot of information about the mentor and particular kids and also thinking about each of their styles. Sometimes, I start to pull all of this together and I think, hey, this mentor could open the door for this particular kid and that would be so wonderful."

Wendy is quick to point out that successful matches also depend on the motivation of the young person and mentor to stick with the relationship even through difficult phases. Every relationship has its rough spots, and mentoring is no exception. Nancy, the mentor we met in Chapter 1, described some of the difficulties and frustrations she encountered with Angela, including several occasions when her protégé actively tried to terminate the relationship. Confused and angry at first, Nancy began to realize that what Angela was looking for was reassurance that she would not be abandoned. "She wanted to know that I really needed her in my life. Which, of course, I desperately did."

Other mentors complain about the everyday frustrations of missed meetings, unreturned phone calls, and backsliding that seems inevitably to follow success. As Wendy contends, "All mentors face some challenges with their Littles [the Big Brothers Big Sisters name for protégés]. Whether or not they stick it out often has to do with how they withstand the stress—a lot of it is simply what the mentors bring to the table." An emerging literature on mentoring styles seems to support these observations. Good interpersonal skills, attentiveness, motivation, and an effort to include youth in decisions are essential, but so is the mentors' persistence in initiating and scheduling consistent meetings.[8]

Caseworkers are typically responsible for monitoring the progress of relationships. Through phone calls and logs they track the match and provide assistance over rough spots. Caseworker involvement varies considerably across programs, ranging from weekly contact to less than one phone call per month. Because the ratio of active matches to caseworkers can be quite high, the amount of time that can be spent on any given match is limited.[9] Nonetheless, ongoing support is often needed to sustain relationships through difficult periods. In fact, across all types of mentoring programs, volunteers who are offered continuing support and supervision are more likely to persist than those who are not contacted regularly by staff.[10]

Support groups consisting of just mentors themselves can play an important role in this process, though they are not an adequate substitute for professional supervision. Approximately 40 percent of mentoring programs have such support groups in place.[11] Other strategies that help sustain relationships include specifying regular meeting times and places and providing the mentor with small stipends and other means to offset the expense of transportation, tickets to movies or other events, snacks and gifts.[12]

Despite careful screening and interviewing, sustained contacts and case management, and even intuition informed by long experience, there is a fair amount of luck involved in determining whether a relationship ends up among the half that flourish or the half that fail. Paired with someone like Walter, Cameron might have thrived; paired with Rick, Patrick might have escalated his fighting. The stakes are high; yet few studies have tried to discover additional indicators that might help case managers identify mentors and youth at high risk for early termination, nor have they examined what aspects of mentoring are most effective and how training might be improved. Instead, many programs have their own, somewhat idiosyncratic, training manuals based on broadly defined notions of how relationships work and how adolescents develop.

Training Manuals

The content of some of the manuals appear to be derived, at least in part from, Public/Private Venture's ongoing research initiative on mentoring programs and from their new training handbook, *The ABCs of School-Based Mentoring*, developed in collaboration with the Northwest Regional Educational Laboratory.[13] This handbook emphasizes careful screening, training, support, and supervision, as do the training manuals of several other organizations (such as The National Mentoring Partnership's *Mentor Training Curriculum* and Big Brothers Big Sisters of America's *Volunteer Education and Development Manual*). Similarly, other research-based mentoring programs, such as Linking Lifetimes, derive their training from empirically validated strategies and place considerable emphasis on sustaining relationships.[14]

As for other programs, the content of their manuals appears to stem largely from the experiences and priorities of the individual program staff rather than from more objective empirical research. These less rigorous approaches often include exhaustive lists of topics to be covered, while providing very little information about how to accomplish these goals. Simply saying that training should include "skills development" is not the same as describing what those skills should be and how they can be developed. There is scant coverage of such topics as how to communicate effectively with teens, how to handle diversity issues, how to anticipate and manage terminations, and so forth.

Why do so many programs minimize volunteer training? Although some leaders might fail to recognize the complexities involved in forming and sustaining relationships with adolescents, for others it may be this very recognition that compels them to forgo in-depth coverage. They may choose instead to put their energy into selecting mentors who possess tried-and-true people skills. And of course many mentors manage to seamlessly connect with adolescents despite having had very little training or supervision. But mentoring does not come easily to everyone, and difficulties sometimes arise that overtax even the most skilled volunteers.

As mentoring continues to expand, it is important to evaluate the training available to volunteers and to optimize those efforts. We need to know more about the core elements of successful mentoring relationships and how these might vary as a function of the needs and characteristics of particular youth. Such issues are complex and tap into the very heart of what constitutes a helping relationship. Although few studies have addressed these issues within the specific context of mentoring relationships, a substantial body of empirical research on helping relationships in counseling and therapeutic settings is relevant. Of course, mentoring and therapy are quite different from each other in many ways, but the commonalties offer some limited insight.

Differences and Similarities between Therapy and Mentoring

The biggest difference between a therapist and a mentor is the professional status of the therapist, which places some constraints on relationships with clients. For example, therapists tend to be highly trained to diagnose and treat emotional disorders. Therapists' activities with clients, meeting times, and venues are more highly circumscribed, and in most cases therapists—unlike mentors—are reimbursed for their professional services. Additionally, while most therapeutic relationships are time-limited and problem-focused, many mentoring relationships have indefinite endpoints and goals. Finally, large caseloads limit the personal investment that a therapist can make in any given relationship, whereas mentors, who have only one protégé, sometimes throw themselves into their relationship with this particular young person.

Despite these and other differences, some common threads run through the two kinds of relationships. For example, both tend to be somewhat removed from the social network of family, friends, and neighbors, yet they are supported by another kind of infrastructure: the therapist's professional community and the volunteer's mentoring program. Both mentoring and therapeutic relationships tend to be hierarchical and involve scheduled "sessions," often on a weekly basis. The most important commonality, however, is that both relationships involve a human connection whose explicit goal is to foster the positive development of one of the partners. When positive change comes about in the client or protégé, it is often the result of an empathic bond with the therapist or mentor.

In the following sections, I will review the research literature on mentoring and therapeutic relationships in an attempt to shed additional light onto the various processes involved in recruiting, screening, matching, training, and supervising mentors.

Recruiting

As mentioned throughout this book, one impediment to creating sustained relationships can be the somewhat cavalier approach that is sometimes taken to recruiting volunteers. At a very basic level, new marketing strategies are needed that accurately describe the benefits a volunteer can expect and the commitment that is required. Some marketing strategies exaggerate the potential benefits of mentoring while downplaying the degree of commitment necessary to achieve these gains. As one administrator conceded, "Given their scarcity, we don't want to scare away potential volunteers. Instead, our hope is that when they connect with a child, they'll get hooked."

One program advertises by asking, "Have you ever thought

about being a mentor? Think about it now. You can do it. It's easier than you think. Sometimes it's work–mostly it's fun." Another popular campaign suggests that volunteers can reverse the lives of troubled adolescents in "less time than you think." Exaggerated marketing campaigns that implore volunteers to be heroic within a relatively short period of time may, in fact, be counterproductive. More humble individuals are likely to feel daunted by what one official humorously referred to as the "Mother Teresa problem." Portraying mentoring as a series of small wins that emerge from an enduring relationship may be more appealing to individuals who want to be helpful but do not necessarily see themselves as miracle workers.

Thus, providing potential volunteers with more accurate information about mentoring could have two positive effects: it could lower the bar to include people with a more humble self-image, while enabling volunteers—including those with a grandiose vision of their ability to make a difference—to make better informed decisions about the necessary commitment, the challenges, and the possible disappointments.

Screening

Once recruited, volunteers should be stringently screened by program staff who are sensitive to any circumstances and characteristics that might put volunteers at risk for early termination.

In our study of mentoring relationships, Jean Grossman and I identified several factors among youth that are predictive of early termination.[15] For example, matches involving 13- to 16-year-olds were 65 percent more likely to terminate in any given month than were matches with 10- to 12-year-olds. This is not surprising, since older adolescents tend to be more peer-oriented than their younger counterparts and less responsive to structured programs. Relationships with adolescents who had been referred for psychological treatment or educational remediation were also less likely to remain intact. These youth may present challenges that overwhelm mentors' capacity or willingness to help.

Similarly, relationships with youth who had sustained emotional, sexual, or physical abuse were more likely to terminate prematurely. The challenges associated with mentoring adolescents who have been maltreated are substantial and, at least in the early stages of the relationship, often accompanied by fewer rewards. Abused youth frequently have more difficulties trusting adults and may have little experience with behaviors that establish and maintain closeness and support.[16] Maltreated youth sometimes expect rejection, and when early terminations happen, they often experience considerable difficulties.[17]

This is not to say that adolescents with these kinds of problems cannot benefit from mentoring. My colleagues and I found that youth in foster homes, many of whom had suffered child abuse and neglect, achieved positive results when they received mentoring.[18] Nonetheless, vulnerable young people appear to be at elevated risk for early termination, and program staff should provide close supervision so that problems can be detected early, possibly in time for a remedy.

Several characteristics of mentors were also predictive of the duration of a mentoring relationship. For example, matches involving volunteers with higher incomes tended to last longer than those involving volunteers with lower incomes. Higher-income mentors probably had greater flexibility in their work schedules and could more readily afford amenities such as childcare and personal transportation that make sustained contact more convenient. Marriage was also a risk factor for early termination. Relative to matches with 18- to 25-year-old volunteers, married volunteers aged 26 to 30 years were 86 percent more likely than average to terminate each month. On the other hand, unmarried volunteers aged 26 to 30 were 65 percent *less* likely to terminate each month.

Although we did not specifically ask about volunteers' families, the competing demands of small children among the married group may have left them with neither the time nor the flexibility needed to sustain contact with potentially troubled youth. By contrast, unmarried adults in their late twenties may have been more open to forming an attachment and may have approached volunteering as an opportunity to meet other volunteers their age, enrich their lives, and contribute to the community—motivations that are associated with mentoring relationships that endure over time.[19]

The gap in age between the mentor and adolescent had no bearing on the length of the relationship. Although caseworkers, parents, and youth sometimes preferred certain age configurations, these preferences did not predict duration.

In addition to screening out or perhaps enhancing support to volunteers who may have difficulty making the necessary commitment, it might also be helpful to tap into pools of volunteers who are likely to stand the test of time. Some programs have recognized the enormous volunteer potential that exists among retired adults, for example. Older adults have more time to devote to this pursuit and are ideally positioned to provide the level of personal attention and emotional support that many youth need. Nearly 30 million Americans (12 percent of the population) are over 65, and this number will double in the next thirty years.[20] Older adults today are enjoying good health and longevity, and often they are looking for part-time volunteer opportunities to keep their bodies and minds active. Those who have experienced marginal status themselves can be quite effective at reaching high-risk youth.[21]

Across Ages, a program developed by Temple University's

Center for Learning, successfully involves older adult volunteers (ranging in age from 60 to 85) who serve as mentors to young people. Remarkably, the pairs spend an average of four to five hours a week together, and the relationships typically endure for many years. Youth in this program engage in less substance use and have better attitudes toward school, the future, and elders over time, as determined by surveys. Additionally, as involvement with mentors went up, truancy declined and behavior in other areas improved.[22]

This is not to say that we should give up on middle-aged or younger adults who are more pressed for time. Sometimes the active adults who are stretched to their limits make the most invigorating role models. These individuals often can connect with adolescents who are less responsive to retired adults, opening opportunities to the working world. This should challenge us to develop strategies and incentives to facilitate the volunteer efforts of working parents and other adults.

For example, organizations that permit their employees to volunteer as mentors during company time can play an important role in facilitating this process. North Carolina State employees receive 24 hours of community-service leave each year, plus 12 additional hours for anyone volunteering in a school. Public school teachers in New York who oversee mentoring programs currently receive a $3,500 stipend for their work. If such efforts were replicated on a national scale, they could go a long way toward addressing the need for committed volunteer mentors and sufficient infrastructure within programs.

Lack of time is not the only impediment to sustained volunteering. For many potential volunteers, a related issue is lack of money. Particularly among people on fixed incomes, such as students and elders, the costs of volunteering may be prohibitive. Many mentors need to arrange childcare and transportation in order to meet with their protégés, and outings often have price tags attached, ranging from the cost of a meal to parking for an event. Although some programs provide mentors with modest stipends and even compensate them for their time, most programs are operating on budgets that preclude such luxuries. Transportation vouchers, on-site childcare, and corporate donations, if taken to a national scale, could sharply reduce the financial burdens of mentoring and give many more people an incentive to volunteer.

Just as not all adults are suited for mentoring, not all youth are suited for being mentored. Although some idealists might argue that every adolescent in this country would benefit from the compassionate attention of a volunteer adult if they had the chance, most realists concede that mentoring cannot substitute for professional treatment among youth who already have serious emotional or behavior problems, nor can it inoculate all youth against developing these problems. Findings from DuBois's recent meta-analysis suggest that mentoring programs are not as effective with adolescents who are struggling with severe difficulties.[23] Grossman and Johnson also found that adolescents overwhelmed by social or behavioral problems were less likely to benefit from mentoring, no matter what style or approach their mentors adopted.[24]

At the other extreme, well-adjusted middle-class youth tend to derive relatively fewer benefits when compared with youth who are facing some degree of difficulty in their lives.[25] Youth who fall in the middle of the continuum of functioning appear most likely to benefit. Furthermore, family and cultural influences may render certain youth less likely to respond to one-on-one mentoring than others. Youth from cultures that emphasize collectivism and deep respect for elders (for example, Native Americans) may be uncomfortable in relationships with unrelated adults. For these youths, more group-oriented approaches may be preferable.[26] Considerable research still needs to be done to determine the parameters of the groups most likely to benefit from mentoring.

Making Matches

Recruiting mentors who are likely to commit to relationships and identifying youth who are most primed to benefit from a mentoring experience are crucial first steps. But they don't automatically lead to matches that click. The critical move is getting mentors and youths together so that they can form first impressions and assess their similarity along a wide range of factors.[27] People tend to make snap judgments about others and then look for information that confirms these first impressions.[28] In most areas of our lives, initial interactions largely determine the nature and success of subsequent encounters. A number of studies of therapy, for example, have demonstrated that the quality of the first few encounters significantly predicts the long-term effectiveness of the relationship.[29]

Similarities between oneself and another person tend to lead to more positive first impressions, so one obvious implication of these findings is that case managers should make matches based on similar interests and backgrounds. Or at least help protégés to identify and build on less obvious commonalities and interests. In a study by Carla Herrera and colleagues, similar interests emerged as one of the most important factors in determining the closeness and supportiveness of the match.[30]

These similarities are not always obvious. One mentor described how she was matched with a nine-year-old girl who was teased by her classmates when she began to wear glasses. According to the volunteer's caseworker, the girl had begun to show signs of diminishing self-esteem and social withdrawal—

such as looking down when she spoke and avoiding interaction. This information led the volunteer, a 28-year-old journalist who normally wears contact lenses, to show up for their first meeting in glasses. "When Jill [her protégée] commented on my glasses, I was able to share my more positive experiences as a child . . . Over the past year we have moved on to many other things, but I still wear my glasses every time!" Other volunteers have described how they connected with their protégés around a range of shared interests (chess, NASCAR, music, bicycle repair) and situations (illness, immigration).

Crossing the Racial Divide

The quest for similarity has led to considerable controversy about cross-race matching. The issue has been studied to some extent in organizational settings and professional helping relationships, but very few studies have directly examined it in the context of youth mentoring.

While some programs take a race-blind approach to matching volunteers with boys and girls, many act on the implicit and sometimes explicit assumption that white mentors (the most common mentor in a cross-race match) cannot appreciate the experiences of minority youth nor fully assist them in achieving their goals. This belief, coupled with the relatively low proportion of minority volunteers (between 15 and 20 percent of all volunteers) and the relatively high proportion of minority youth participants (approximately 50 percent), has resulted in thousands of minority youth being retained on long wait lists until adult volunteers of the same race become available.[31] What are the pros and cons of cross-race versus same-race matching? What light can the research literature shed on this sensitive topic?

Proponents of same-race matches believe that mentors with a similar racial and ethnic background are better equipped to understand the social and psychological conflicts of minority youth and to share deep levels of trust and cooperation with their protégés. The sense of guilt and defensiveness that white mentors may experience as they confront racial oppression could hinder their capacity to address issues of central importance to minorities.[32] Similarly, minority adolescents may feel particularly sensitive to being judged by white mentors according to negative stereotypes, and that fear may discourage these youths from making the effort and taking the risks that could potentially bolster their self-esteem.[33] Finally, pairing white mentors with minority adolescents may undermine the adolescents' sense of cultural identity or convey a message that appropriate role models are to be found in their own group.[34]

Many of those who defend cross-race matching do not deny the potential effects of culture and race on mentoring relationships. But they are troubled by the notoriously long wait lists facing many minority youth, and they believe that effective relationships can develop despite racial, ethnic, and class differences.[35] Ronald Ferguson, for example, found evidence of positive cross-race relationships in several mentoring programs. He noted that although "several people had strong opinions about the need for matching children and mentors by sex and race . . . sensitivity seems to be the only absolute requirement."[36]

Melanie Morrow and Kristen Styles found that effective relationships were just as likely to form in cross-race pairs as in same-race pairs.[37] Although challenges arose due to the cultural differences, they were generally resolved through adequate support and understanding. These findings are consistent with those of Herrera and colleagues, who found that cross-race matches were as close and supportive as same-race matches and that other factors (such as type of activities, shared interests, and mentor training) accounted for far more of the variance in quality than did racial identification.[38]

Some researchers see socioeconomic status as more of a concern than issues of race or ethnicity.[39] Erwin Flaxman and colleagues noted that in settings where middle-class adults are attempting to work with urban adolescents, the mentors' world can easily seem "irrelevant or even nonsensical" to youth, "and their goals for mentees naïve."[40] Finally, some claim that cross-race matching, rather than being a disadvantage, can actually bridge social distances and challenge negative stereotypes. Through positive connections with white mentors, minority adolescents may begin to perceive supportive aspects of the white community, which are often overshadowed by perceived or very real racism.[41]

My colleagues and I recently looked at the issue of same-race versus cross-race relationships.[42] Our study focused on 476 youth in the Big Brothers Big Sisters national survey (approximately half of the overall sample were members of minority groups). All of the cross-race volunteer mentors were white. Mentors in same-race and cross-race matches were similar at the study's outset, except that minority volunteers were more likely to have children living at home. Minority youth in the two groups did not differ on any of the outcome variables at the beginning of the study.

When we examined 16 outcome variables at the end of the study, only one group difference stood out: adolescents in same-race matches were somewhat more likely to report the initiation of alcohol use than adolescents in cross-race matches. However, a scattering of findings emerged when the groups were further differentiated by gender. Minority boys in cross-race matches experienced a slightly greater decline in perceived scholastic competence and self-worth than minority boys in same-race matches. Minority girls in cross-race matches experienced greater declines in the value they placed on school and self-worth than minority girls in same-race matches.

Youth in the two groups held relatively similar impressions of their mentors. Those in cross-race matches, however, reported feeling that they could more often "talk to their mentors" when things were bothering them and that they received more unconditional support. Finally, parents and guardians held somewhat more positive impressions of cross-race relationships. In particular, parents of youth in cross-race matches were more likely than parents of youth in same-race matches to report that the relationships led to improvements in their children's peer relationships, that the mentors built on their children's strengths, and that the mentors provided recreational and social opportunities. These findings converge with the youths' own qualitative assessments and suggest that cross-race mentors may be working particularly hard to overcome the challenges of crossing racial boundaries.

This sparse array of inconsistent findings suggests that the racial configuration of a match, per se, does not affect the outcomes for the youth in any consistent manner. Indeed, the fact that most of the group differences emerged only after the groups were further differentiated by gender suggests that the effects of race on relationships are subtle and act in combination with other factors, such as gender, interpersonal style, and parental attitudes, to shape the mentoring experience. With the exception of youth for whom racial issues are an overriding concern, the mentor's race or ethnicity may not be the critical factor in predicting the likelihood of a successful relationship.

The study did not include measures of cultural pride, which may have been influenced by the mentors' race.

Trusting and supportive relationships appear to be possible for minority youth in both same-race and cross-race relationships, and the quality of these relationships appears to be multi-determined. In the following section, I will review what is known about predicting the quality of relationships and the implications of this knowledge for training mentors.

Building Strong Relationships

After screening and matching take place, the next challenge for program staff is to help mentors and youth foster a strong bond. As mentioned in Chapter 2, the strength of this bond often determines the impact of the relationship. When data from the national evaluation of Big Brothers Big Sisters were reanalyzed to control for relationship quality, those who gave their mentors the highest positive ratings derived far more benefits than those who gave their mentors more negative ratings.[43]

Herrera and colleagues examined the predictors of mentoring relationship quality, interviewing 669 volunteers who were in one-on-one matches in community and school-based programs.[44] Relationship quality was measured by the degree of closeness; the emotional support provided—the extent to which mentors are "always there" for protégés and show them that they care about what happens to them; and the instrumental support—the extent to which mentors help protégés "improve at some particular skill" and feel empowered to "take a chance at doing something new." These factors were chosen because in previous studies they have been associated with longer-lasting relationships, positive outcomes for youth, and greater mentor satisfaction.[45] Researchers supplemented mentor data with interviews and focus groups conducted with youth, school, and agency staff. The study revealed several factors that were important in determining the quality of relationships in both community and school-based programs.

The strongest contributing factor to all three measures of relationships was the extent to which the youth and mentors engaged in social activities (for example, having lunch, just hanging out together). Other relationship factors that predicted close relationships were engaging in academic activities, meeting more than ten hours per month, and joint decision making. Four program practices also predicted strong relationships: making matches based on similar interests; providing more than six hours of volunteer training; offering post-match training and support; and reasonably intensive screening.

Along similar lines, my students and I recently analyzed a range of mentor relationships and then systematically measured associations between types of relationships and youth outcomes.[46] The study, which drew on data from the national evaluation of Big Brothers Big Sisters, focused on the protégés' responses to 56 questions designed to assess how the frequency and type of activities that mentors participated in with their protégés affected protégés' feelings toward their mentors. Youth who characterized their relationships as providing moderate levels of activity and structure derived the largest number of benefits when compared with the control group—including lower levels of alienation from parents, less conflict and inequality with friends, and higher levels of self-worth and school competence. By contrast, youth who characterized their mentors as being highly supportive but providing relatively few opportunities for structured activity derived the fewest benefits. Consistent with previous work, these findings underscore the importance of involvement in enjoyable activities. As Sipe concluded, "Not only is having fun a key part of relationship-building, but it provides youth with opportunities that are often not otherwise available to them."[47]

Taken together, these findings touch on broader debates in the field over the best approach to establishing a good connection with an adolescent. Some researchers suggest that close relationships are most likely to emerge as the by-product of shared involvement in social, academic, career, or other activities. Darling, Hamilton, and Niego, for example, have argued that mentors who engage with youth in challenging, goal-directed activities are more likely to be successful than those whose primary focus is to get to know the adolescent. They note that emotional relationships grow out of adults' validation of adolescents' effort and ability. "Ironically, relationships were built when building a relationship was not the main purpose of getting together."[48]

Others have highlighted the importance of taking the lead from adolescents themselves, in a more emotion-focused approach.[49] McClanahan, for example, found that youth who were engaged in more emotionally based activities reported more positive perceptions of their relationships than those whose relationships focused primarily on working toward goals.[50]

Gender differences come into play here as well. Cambridge Big Brothers program director John Pearson observed that "on average, the typical Big Sister might sit down and talk—that's the *last* thing guys want to do! They are going to go do something, and if they happen to talk while they are doing it, well that's a very good sign." Others see this difference less in terms of gender than in terms of the interpersonal styles and interests of each adolescent. For example, younger adolescents, whose levels of cognitive sophistication leave them less inclined to engage in abstract conversations, may instead gravitate more toward more structured activities.[51]

Of course, good mentors take their cues from their protégés to strike a comfortable balance among having fun, working toward practical goals, and exploring emotions. Mentors must try to be sensitive to their protégés' circumstances and input and calibrate their approach accordingly. Margaret Beam and colleagues noted that more than 80 percent of adults whom adolescents described as being "very important" to them were perceived to have some combination of the following traits: providing emotional support, showing respect for the adolescent, offering availability as someone to talk to, and supporting the adolescent's engagement in activities.[52]

Researchers have highlighted other approaches of successful mentors, including consistency, respecting the youth's viewpoints, and seeking supervision from support staff when needed. Successful mentors tended to become acquainted, yet not overly involved, with their protégés' families and tended to respect the youths' desire to have fun. Echoing these conclusions, Grossman and Johnson found stronger beneficial effects among pairs who interacted more frequently and in which mentors sought the input of the youth and took a more open, less judgmental stance with them.[53] Additionally, Hendrey, Rogers, Glendinning, and Coleman found that the mentors' capacity to refrain from harsh judgement, effectively cope with difficulties, and express optimism and confidence made important contributions to the mentoring relationships.[54]

These findings have implications for the selection and training of volunteer mentors. Effective relationships emerge, it seems, through a combination of structure, activity, and emotional support, a mix calibrated in response to the needs of the particular adolescent and the stage of the relationship.

Benchmarks of Effective Relationships

It would be nice if a reasonably short questionnaire that protégés could fill out would provide an ongoing gauge of the health and effectiveness of a relationship. To see if such a tool could be designed, my colleagues and I recently reanalyzed responses to a 71-item questionnaire, on which protégés in the national survey were asked to characterize their mentor relationships.[55] We used factor analysis to statistically determine the ways in which individual items on a questionnaire group together to measure an underlying factor or characteristic.

Four factors, encompassing 15 items in the survey, stood out as ways to distinguish between successful and unsuccessful relationships: Is the relationship helpful? Does it meet expectations? Does it evoke negative emotions? And does the protégé feel close to the mentor? (see Table 1).[56] Successful and enduring mentoring relationships tended to be defined less in terms of mentors' positive virtues or any particular activities they engaged in than by the absence of disappointing characteristics. For example, over 50 of the positively-framed items (for example, "When I am with my mentor I feel happy, I look forward to seeing my mentor") held no predictive power. Instead, it was often the absence of negatively framed items ("When I am with my mentor I feel disappointed") that predicted outcomes.

Although somewhat disconcerting, these findings underscore the damaging effects of disappointment and mistrust in mentoring relationships and are consistent with findings that have emerged in the social support literature on the relatively larger impact of negative, versus positive, interactions.[57] Taken

Table 1. The Mentor Questionnaire

1. When something is bugging me, my mentor listens to me while I get it off my chest.
2. My mentor has lots of good ideas about how to solve a problem.
3. My mentor helps me take my mind off things by doing something with me.
4. Sometimes my mentor promises that we will do something and then we don't do it.
5. My mentor makes fun of me in ways that I don't like.
6. I wish my mentor was different.
7. When I am with my mentor, I feel disappointed.
8. When I am with my mentor, I feel ignored.
9. When I am with my mentor, I feel bored.
10. When I am with my mentor, I feel mad.
11. I feel that I can't trust my mentor with secrets because I am afraid s/he would tell my parent/guardian.
12. When my mentor gives me advise, s/he makes me feel kind of stupid.
13. I wish my mentor asked me more about what I think.
14. I wish my mentor knew me better.
15. I wish my mentor spent more time with me.

*Responses for items 1–3 range from hardly ever (1) to pretty often (4); responses for 4–15 range from very true (1) to not at all true (4).

together these 15 items could be administered periodically to protégés as a metric of relationship quality.

Comparisons with Findings about Therapy

As described in Chapter 2, a solid, collaborative alliance between a therapist and a client is a crucial ingredient in any therapeutic approach.[58] Several attitudes and behaviors on the part of the therapist contribute to the quality of this alliance. Empathy, respect, receptivity, non-judgmental listening, not attacking the client's dignity, and not minimizing or dismissing problems are important to all clients, irrespective of the particular therapeutic approach.[59] The therapist's level of experience does not appear to influence the strength of the relationship; therapists and paraprofessionals can be equally effective.[60] Warmth, support, and self-disclosure on the part of the therapist seems to vary as a crucial factor, depending on the client—a fact which highlights the importance of flexibility on the part of the therapist in responding to a client's needs and expectations at various phases of the relationship.[61]

Several characteristics of clients have also been identified as crucially important to maintaining the quality of the therapist-client bond. Motivation, involvement, and cooperation in therapy, as well as an openness to issues and emotions, are seen as important predictors of the quality of the therapeutic relationship and of a positive outcome for the client.[62] On the other hand, prolonged defensiveness and hostility on the part of the client has been shown to impede the development of a sound working relationship.[63] Alexandra Bachelor has pointed out that many clients underestimate the importance of their own participation and place full responsibility for the relationship with the therapist.[64] This attitude does not maximize the chances that the therapy will be successful.

These findings could have implications for how protégés are screened for mentoring programs. From the onset, protégés should be provided with realistic expectations regarding what their mentors can (and cannot) do, and their own role in maintaining the relationship should be emphasized. They should be encouraged to take active ownership of the process. Although some youth may be initially passive or even resistant, with case management and mentor perseverance they might become more cooperative and take more initiative. Nonetheless, mentors should remain sympathetic to the fact that some adolescents in mentoring programs have weathered difficulties and separations in their other important relationships in their lives, and this complicates their capacity to form trusting bonds with mentors.

Providing Supervision

Case managers should help sensitize mentors to adolescents' needs and expectations and should attempt to anticipate problems that might arise. Susan Murphy and Ellen Ensher described mentoring relationships as progressing through five general phases:

- Introductions: Participants look for similarities and make judgments.
- Relationship building: Protégé and mentor engage in positive activities that give them things to talk about and remember and opportunities to spend time together.
- Growth: Through relatively open communication and role modeling, the mentor provides emotional and instrumental support to the protégé.
- Maturation: The pair focus on the protégés' goals, and mentors begin to derive benefits as well.
- Transition: The relationship declines or is redefined.[65]

These stages can serve as a compass for case managers to gauge their level of involvement, predict periods of instability, and assess progress. Program staff can draw on their knowledge of the phases of relationships to interpret and effectively respond to common patterns of protégé behavior.

For example, caseworkers often describe a sequence in which adolescents in relatively new relationships sometimes make a dramatic "leap to health" in their attitudes and behaviors, followed by a setback and an unraveling of earlier gains.

The setback often coincides with the transition from "Relationship building" to "Growth." This is the point when mentors begin to leverage the trust and good will that has been built up to focus on points of vulnerability. This stage can be unsettling to protégés, who may begin to miss meetings or withdraw from discussions. As one program staff member observed, "Relationships usually get off to a pretty good start, with the mentor bending over backwards for the kid, but there is usually a turning point where things get more intense. How this is handled can make all the difference in whether the relationship deepens or falls apart." Case managers can play an important role in helping mentors and adolescents understand setbacks and maintain or restore momentum.

Case managers can also help the mentor and youth calibrate their expectations. Both parties are likely to have preconceptions about the relationship that influence how they judge one another over its course. One of the tasks of a caseworker should be to challenge unrealistic expectations and to gauge feelings over time. For example, mentors should be encouraged to identify their feelings toward their protégés. This self-analysis can be facilitated by discussions with caseworkers that focus on earlier experiences in the mentors' own lives that drew them into the helping role.

Although the mentoring experience permits closeness and empathy that can be extraordinarily helpful to struggling adolescents, it can also create vulnerabilities in the adult. Mentors experience a host of emotions throughout the course of their volunteer work with young people. Even the most dedicated mentors are likely to feel exasperation, ambivalence, anger, and regret at various points. Programs that validate such reactions as they arise and openly acknowledge the emotional costs of volunteering throughout the duration of the relationship may help mentors keep relationships with their protégés alive.

Handling Terminations

Research on early terminations in therapy, including the specific behaviors and attitudes that increase their likelihood, is relevant to mentoring relationships. Nearly half of all therapeutic ties terminate prematurely, owing to a variety of factors.[66] Sometimes parents or spouses sabotage the process; sometimes clients reenact earlier, dysfunctional behaviors; and sometimes clients are dissatisfied with their therapists or feel disappointed with how therapy is progressing. Clients rarely tell their therapists when they are upset with the process, preferring instead to withdraw from direct confrontation.[67]

Changes in therapists' circumstances, such as relocations, illnesses, graduations, new jobs, or childbirth, can also precipitate terminations. When the end of a therapeutic relationship is initiated by the therapist, it can be very destructive to adolescents' sense of well-being. Donald Winnicott noted that adolescence is a "very awkward time" for therapists to prematurely end treatment given adolescents' physical, cognitive, and socioemotional transitions. Cathy Siebold also warned that, "termination by the therapist confounds the typical clinical course and breaks an essential rule of therapy—that the therapist will tolerate, survive, and encourage the patient's continued attendance and communication."[68]

Similar challenges precipitate premature terminations in mentoring. Mentors and protégés bring complex personal histories to the table that can interact in countless ways, some of which may destroy any chances of a bond developing between them. Case managers should be sensitive to factors that might place the relationship at risk and cognizant of the fact that protégés are unlikely to lodge complaints in response to the inadequacies of their mentors.

Nonetheless, the research literature on therapeutic terminations offers some insights into effective strategies for minimizing difficulties.[69] Despite the similarities, the meaning and context of terminations in therapy and mentoring differ. Many mentoring relationships, particularly those that are focused on specific academic or career goals, never develop the level of intensity that characterizes therapeutic ties, and other relationships are time-limited by design.

When Mentors Terminate a Relationship

Mentors who anticipate an impending termination should give their protégés ample warning. A few weeks' notice and an appropriately detailed explanation can provide adolescents with a better understanding, reassurances, and the opportunity to reach some sort of closure. Unfortunately, mentors are often reluctant to broach the topic and often postpone discussions. They may feel guilty and fearful of negative reactions.

Styles and Morrow found that terminations by male mentors tended to be less complicated and hurtful than those of female mentors. Male mentors tended to provide ample warning and to offer clear and direct explanations for their actions. Female mentors tended to be more reluctant, opting to gradually withdraw rather than discuss the issue forthrightly. Although women acted out of feelings of guilt and a desire to protect their protégés' feelings, their less straightforward approach sent mixed messages and heightened feelings of loss on the part of the protégés.[70]

A mentor's departure might evoke memories of other losses and ignite painful and confusing feelings. Writing of therapist-initiated terminations, Paul Dewald warned that they "may be perceived as a repetition of arbitrary, unexpected and 'selfish' behavior of earlier key figures, particularly when there have been significant or traumatic separations earlier in the patient's life"; similar findings can hold true for mentor-initiated terminations. In the case of therapist-initiated terminations, Dewald observed that a patient's response would usually be consistent with reactions to similar previous situations.[71]

Adolescents' reactions to the termination of mentoring vary considerably, and few feel devastated by their mentor's departure. Nonetheless, mentors should be prepared to address feelings of hurt, even when they are not immediately apparent, and to share their own feelings of loss. Case managers can help mentors anticipate negative reactions and rehearse strategies for handling them. In some instances it may be advisable for the mentor to meet with the protégé infrequently for a period of time after the official termination or to transfer the protégé to a new mentor.

Transferring to a New Mentor

Although transferring protégés to new mentors is common practice in many programs, the process can be more psychologically complex than it appears. That is certainly the case for therapist transfers. Anna Freud suggested that "it is generally advisable for a patient who must terminate with one therapist to wait and only later start again with another therapist if necessary."[72] Although this advice might not always apply to mentoring, it does underscore the importance of not simply replacing the mentor with another before adequate closure on the first relationship has been reached. The caseworker should attempt to understand and address the reasons for the first termination so as to minimize the likelihood of repeating a dysfunctional pattern. This can be tricky, particularly when a mentor has terminated in response to feeling overwhelmed by the youth's difficult circumstances or neediness. When appropriate, youth should be helped to learn from dysfunctional patterns of relating so as to reduce the likelihood that they will be repeated.

When Protégés Terminate a Relationship

Although I highlighted a mentor-initiated termination in Chapter 3, it is sometimes the protégé who puts an end to things. Some adolescents might present the termination as a fait accompli, while others broach the subject more tentatively. An adolescent's stated desire to end the relationship should not always be taken at face value, however. As many mentors can attest, threatening to end the relationship is a very effective way for youth to signal discontent. Once it is clear, however, that the youth is determined to leave, the mentor should not attempt to strongly influence the decision.

Some youth withdraw from the relationship by not responding to phone calls or chronically standing up their mentors. These sorts of default terminations can sometimes be avoided when mentors and caseworkers pick up on cues that might signal a protégé's disengagement (for example, frequent lateness, missed meetings, and distracted, perfunctory responses to open-ended questions). Youth sometimes withdraw because they feel better, or because the relationship has progressed to a more emotionally challenging level. Still others might fear that they are letting their mentors down and chose to withdraw from the relationship rather than face their mentors' disappointment.

Whatever the reason, exploring and evaluating a protégé's reason to terminate can be a delicate process. Mentors should talk with caseworkers to become aware of their own feelings of sadness, anger, rejection, and, in some instances, relief. This awareness will enable mentors to more openly discuss the impending termination with their protégés.

Termination Activities

Regardless of whether the termination was scheduled or unscheduled, and irrespective of who might have initiated it, activities can be a useful means of involving the protégé in the termination process. These activities, which were adapted in part from literature on terminations in child psychotherapy, can help mentors and protégés review the relationship, highlight accomplishments, address issues of loss, and reframe the ending. For example, mentors can help their protégés anticipate and gain some sense of control over the end of the relationship by jointly making a calendar or a picture of an hourglass that signifies remaining meetings, or creating a timeline in which the termination date is set. Activities that address loss might include sharing photographs of the mentor and protégé together, or making hand drawings, in which the mentor's hand is outlined next to the adolescent's. The mentor can also work with the protégé to make a memory box or collage that depicts feelings, skills, and memories of shared activities. Finally, the mentor and protégé should work together to plan a special fun outing prior to the final meeting.

In summary, all terminations, even planned ones that follow successful relationships, can evoke conflicting emotions and defensive reactions. The termination is an influential piece of the entire mentoring process that is not given adequate attention in many training programs. How relationships end, however, can color the ways that protégés think about their entire experience. In addition to preventing feelings of abandonment and loss, a well-handled termination can provide a healthy model for sharing feelings around other losses in adolescents' lives.

A Word of Warning

There will always be some degree of mystery in determining what makes two people click. But just as researchers of romantic ties have uncovered some of the reasons two people fall and stay in love, greater specificity in mentoring can only help in the matching and maintenance of relationships.[73] In this chapter, research on therapeutic relationships has been brought to bear on mentoring. Additional recommendations can be found on websites such as www.mentoring.org, www.nwrel.org/mentoring, www.bbbsa.org, and www.ed.gov/pubs/YesYouCan as well as in program materials and The National Mentoring Partnership's widely distributed guide, *Mentoring: Elements of Effective Practice*.

Although the mentoring guidelines presented here and elsewhere are useful, an individual approach to each youth should be crafted. As Penelope Leach wrote in her parenting guide, "Rearing a child 'by the book'—by any set of rules or predetermined ideas—can work well if the rules you choose to follow fit the [child] you happen to have. But even a minor misfit between the two can cause misery."[74] Frequent contact with experienced and knowledgeable caseworkers can help inexperienced mentors find the right balance of approaches for their protégés.

Guidelines can only touch the surface of the intricacies involved in mentoring someone. As Robert Coles warned, "A handbook of do's and don'ts and how-to's and how-not-to's [cannot] spare us the ironies and complexities and inconsistencies of human nature as they connect with the experience known as service."[75]

Thus, the guidelines and suggestions that are presented here and elsewhere are likely to be most effective when they are used not as a formulaic approach but as a framework that leaves room for volunteers' intuitive wisdom. These guidelines should be incorporated with a spirit of self-reflection, perseverance, and openness to the particular circumstances and style of one's protégé. This includes a willingness to serve not only as a model for the adolescent but also as someone who is genuine and has flaws. As Rabbi Zalman Schacter-Shalomi and Ronald Miller recommend in their book *From Age-ing to Sage-ing:* "Listen with great spaciousness of heart and mind to your mentee's genuine concerns before attempting to share your wisdom; don't impose but evoke your mentee's innate knowing; don't try to impress your mentee by claiming to be perfect; be your searching, tentative, very human self instead; respect and call forth your mentee's uniqueness; recognize that like everything else under the sun, mentoring has its seasons."[76]

5

Mentoring in Perspective

> Mentoring is like finding a gusher or having invested in America Online at the beginning; we should applaud its success, and use it for all its worth.
>
> Gary Walker, President of Public/Private Ventures

In the early 1990s Marc Freedman, author of *The Kindness of Strangers*, worried that the rapid expansion of mentoring programs in the absence of sufficient guidelines and resources had amounted to "fervor without infrastructure."[1] A decade later this fervor has reached an even higher pitch. A visit to the many websites devoted to the topic provides ample indication of mentoring's popularity. At a recent mentoring conference, many participants spoke of "bringing mentoring to scale" and of "growing mentoring" so that virtually every school or community has a program in place.

Although Freedman's prescient warnings continue to ring true, the good news is that far more infrastructure sustain mentoring efforts today than just a decade ago. As mentoring programs have continued to expand, national mentoring organizations have flourished into a rich network of support. Although these organizations sometimes compete for turf in ways that are counterproductive to their collective goals and occasionally engage in rhetoric that emphasizes quantity over quality, they are infusing programs with important training materials, resources, and organizational ties.

Increased funding to support and sustain mentoring programs is available through a widening array of federal, state, and foundation sources. For example, the Juvenile Mentoring Program (JUMP) at the Office of Juvenile Justice and Delinquency Prevention (OJJDP) received $16 million in appropriations for the fiscal year 2001 to support one-on-one mentoring programs with at-risk youth. The House of Representatives recently passed the Mentoring for Success Act as an amendment to the Elementary and Secondary Education Act. This amendment, which is awaiting Senate approval, would enlist the Department of Education in making grants to local mentoring programs through a $30 million allocation in fiscal year 2002.

Although promising, this funding is still meager when balanced against the number of mentoring programs. Even the most optimistic calculations amount to far less than what is needed to sustain a large number of high-quality relationships in each state. There is also the danger that opportunistic providers may develop programs in response to funding opportunities rather than out of a sincere interest in establishing enduring relationships. Similarly, freestanding programs that rely on single funding sources sometimes fail to sustain themselves beyond the life of a particular grant, leaving mentors and youth in the lurch.

Nonetheless, enhanced resources are likely to continue to improve infrastructure in positive ways. Proposed legislation in New York State would offer certification, based on knowledge and experience, to professionals who run mentoring programs. Efforts are underway to alleviate the barriers to conducting costly background checks on volunteers. The proposed National Child Protection Volunteer Screening Assistance Act would authorize $80 million to establish a clearinghouse where all nonprofit volunteer organizations could request free national criminal background checks.

University-based researchers have shown a heightened interest in developing and evaluating programs that focus on youths' strengths and potential.[2] The growing research attention to positive youth development, the ubiquitous campus-based service learning programs, and the increased number of university-community alliances are all evidence of this trend. College students are flocking to volunteer activities in unprecedented numbers and filling the ranks of mentors in community and school-based settings. The transitory nature of this population can sometimes undermine continuity, but with adequate training and support some of these difficulties can be alleviated. Moreover, early volunteering is the best predictor of lifelong volunteering; so increased involvement among college students has implications for the future viability of mentoring programs and other volunteer community services.[3]

Research and Evaluation

Beyond this direct service component, the growing number of university-community collaborations is likely to result in more program evaluations that can address the fundamental issues that remain unresolved in the field. Careful program evaluations anchored in theory and empirical evidence can contribute to a more theoretically informed and practically applicable understanding of mentoring.

Researchers should assess both the positive and the unintended negative influences of mentoring. For example, although few researchers have considered the siblings of protégés, it is not difficult to imagine the feelings of hurt and jealously that might arise when one member of a family is singled out for opportunities and rewards. The same holds true of parents, who may feel marginalized by their children's relationships with other caring adults. Additionally, high levels of protégé competence, in otherwise low-achieving settings, can create problems with peers and lead to considerable distress.[4]

When Angela—the protégé we met in Chapter 1—began to excel academically, she was accused by peers of "selling out," and she felt increasingly alienated in her school. Her frustrations and doubts eventually escalated into fistfights and a subsequent suspension from school. Suniya Luthar has noted similar patterns among low-income inner-city adolescents—those who are highly competent by external criteria, such as grades and conduct, may experience considerable distress.[5] Research designs that include comparisons among groups on a wide range of variables prior to and following the mentoring program will permit researchers to assess unanticipated positive and negative changes.

It will also be important to develop evaluation strategies to capture the full range of program effects, including those that may be masked by the wide variation across programs and within the treatment groups. Identifying the sources of this variation will help to illuminate elements of effective practice. Additionally, systematic comparisons of programs that vary in type, intensity, supervision, training, matching, and length should be conducted in order to provide a sound basis for comparisons and for decision making in the field. Along these lines, researchers assess both the statistical and practical significance of their findings.[6] Of course, evaluations of treatment effects in mentoring are complicated by the fact that the relationships do not exist in a vacuum and programs are often linked to a broader array of services.

In addition to comparing programs and specifying outcomes, we need a deeper understanding of mentoring relationships. Qualitative studies, as exemplified by the work of Kristine Morrow and Melanie Styles, should continue to be conducted.[7] And brief, empirically validated questionnaires that measure relationship characteristics, such as the one presented in Chapter 4, should be included in evaluations of mentoring programs.[8] Research that captures the reciprocal nature of the mentoring process as it unfolds between the two individuals involved is also needed.[9] Adequate attention to multiple perspectives on the relationship, to the adolescents' developmental phase and approach to the relationship, to cultural diversity, and to the stage of the relationship are needed. Statistical methods that capture the ways in which individual and relationship characteristics contribute to different pathways of development will help to illuminate the processes of change.[10] Marc Freedman observed that "mentoring is mostly about small victories as subtle change." Our challenge will be to develop evaluation strategies that can capture such changes.

Chapter 2 presented a conceptual framework that portrays a close relationship as the catalyst for several intertwined developmental processes. This and related frameworks should be refined through additional research that delves into how, and in what sequence, these processes unfold in different youth. It will be important to examine the ways in which mentor relationships operate within and depart from the emotional frameworks developed through parent-child relationships. Attention to contextual factors, such as family histories and demographic characteristics, might help to explain continuities and discontinuities in adolescents' approach to mentoring relationships.[11]

We should also deepen our understanding of adolescents' vulnerabilities to disruptions. It remains unclear whether the negative effects of terminations that emerged in our study of the duration of relationships stemmed from youths' feelings of rejection and disappointment or from other possible influences. Future studies should include measures of adolescents' sensitivity to rejection, their attributions of mentors' intent, and other factors that might explain this link between early termination and poor outcomes. We should explore adults' motivations for engaging in relationships with unrelated adolescents, the effects of these motivations on commitment to the relationship, and, importantly, the influence of relationships on mentors. Methods that move beyond the individual mentor or protégé are needed to capture the larger context in which relationships unfold. As our society becomes increasingly multicultural, it is ever more important to uncover the processes that contribute to healthy adaptation in adolescents from diverse backgrounds.

Scholarly attention to the processes that govern nonparent adult relationships, and the contexts that give rise to them, could shed additional light onto the many topics that have been raised in this book and bring credibility to the study of nonparent adult relationships that is commensurate with their influence. As Robert Pianta concluded, "Relationships with adults are a cornerstone of development—they are responsible for a large proportion of school success. Too often, the role of the adult-child relationship is underestimated either because it is not well understood or because the role of the context is not understood or emphasized in prevailing models for understanding development."[12]

The analytic toolbox that has deepened our understanding of early parent-child relationships should be brought to bear on a wider range of influential ties. Given that funders and researchers are increasingly turning their gaze toward positive youth development across diverse relationships and settings, we have reason for optimism on this front.

Site-Based Mentoring

Another promising trend, with direct implications for both cost and program infrastructure, is the growing interest in site-based mentoring. Approximately 45 percent of mentoring programs are site-based, with more than 70 percent located in schools and the remaining 30 percent in workplace, agency, and religious settings. Nearly 300,000 school-based matches have been made by Big Brothers Big Sisters agencies alone. School-based programs tend to be about half as costly per youth, even when adding the value of in-kind school contributions. Beyond the cost savings, there appear to be several benefits to school-based mentoring. For example, schools are better able to capitalize on the knowledge, referrals, supervision, and support of the many adults who are already in the setting. This simplifies the program staff's task of forming and monitoring relationships, and there is some preliminary evidence that they can positively affect academic outcomes.[13]

School-based mentoring programs tend to attract volunteers who—by virtue of their jobs, families, age, or other circumstances—are less likely to volunteer in community-based programs. Many companies have partnerships with schools that provide natural linkages, staff incentives, sanctioned leaves, and accountability. Since the weekly meetings typically occur on school grounds, safety concerns are allayed.[14] A recent evaluation of school-based mentoring at five different Big Brothers Big Sisters agencies revealed promising trends, including improved academic performance and better relationships with teachers.[15]

A downside of school-based programs is their link to the academic calendar. Many suspend or even terminate service during summer months. This is shortsighted, particularly since program effects tend to accrue with time, and many behavioral problems and difficulties arise during the summer months. Robert Aseltine and his colleagues recently found that the benefits of a school-based mentoring program did not persist beyond the duration of the school year.[16]

Even during the school year, relationships tend be less intensive than their community-based counterparts.[17] School-based mentors spend about half as much time with youth as community-based mentors (6 hours per month, compared with 12), and the school-based structure tends to constrain the intensity and scope of meetings in ways that community-based relationships do not. Adolescents' needs for comfort and disclosure cannot always be contained neatly within the parameters of a class schedule, and there are limits to what some youth will reveal on school premises. Moreover, school-based mentors' tendency to focus on academics often comes at the expense of the kinds of social activities that help to build close bonds. Not surprisingly, Sipe and colleagues found that significantly more community-based mentors felt "very close" to their protégés than did school-based and work-based mentors (45 percent versus 32 percent, respectively).[18]

These constraints, although considerable, should not discourage what could be a promising response to the infrastructure problems facing community-based programs. A challenge will be to determine how to meld the flexibility, intensity, and enduring nature of successful community-based approaches with the structure and support of school-based approaches.

Taken together, these trends of improved infrastructure and funding, university involvement, and site-based mentoring suggest that we are moving in the right direction, at least with regard to program sustainability, evaluation, and organization. The most pressing challenges concern how best to develop and sustain productive relationships. This territory is subtle and complex and rests on research aimed at analyzing the very nature of human relationships. In essence, basic and applied research efforts need to be brought to bear on the enormous public relations and program efforts that are already under way.

The Limits of Mentoring

Although research that illuminates the complexities of the mentoring relationship will help to improve the effectiveness of programs, mentoring will never be equipped to address the needs of all youth. For one thing, youth are often turned away from over-subscribed mentoring programs or placed on long wait lists. This suggests that mentoring programs do not have the capacity to reach all adolescents who are referred. But even if they could, mentoring programs are not for everyone. Youth who are struggling with even moderately high levels of psychological, behavioral, or social difficulties might be more appropriately referred to professional support.

Unfortunately, mentoring relationships are too often construed as troubled youth's best hope for salvation. For example, President George W. Bush said in his 2001 Inaugural Address, "Some needs and hurts are so deep they will only respond to a mentor's touch or a pastor's prayer." The fact is, however, that the deepest needs of American adolescents are unlikely to be redressed solely by a mentor. Even among higher functioning youth, one-on-one mentoring programs may be unnecessary, inappropriate, or simply too awkward and contrived for their tastes.

Given these constraints, it might be effective in some cases to encourage youth to recruit support from helpful adults in their own social networks. Potential mentors already exist in extended families, schools, churches, neighborhoods, and community organizations, but adolescents are often hesitant to approach them. Rather than creating relationships between strangers, programs can encourage adolescents to cultivate these latent ties.[19] Mentors from within youth's extended reach may be more familiar with the cultural norms, circumstances, and constraints of the setting and better positioned to offer credible advice. Even if such relationships fail to thrive, they are less likely to disappear entirely, potentially offsetting the negative feelings associated with assigned mentor terminations.[20]

Unfortunately, even when youth want to find mentors on their own, settings are often structured in ways that discourage contact with adults. In Chapter 1 we looked at several factors that have conspired to render nonparent adults far less available to youth than they were just a few decades ago. Before we start teaching youth to fish for mentors on any sort of a mass scale, it is important to stock the ponds. At the most immediate level, public policies and institutions have an increasingly important role to play in supporting parents in their efforts to provide more guidance to their own children and adolescents. Greater flexibility in parents' work lives would afford them more time for their children. Community-based family support centers and other publicly-sponsored efforts can help to bring adolescents and related adults together and reinforce the critical role of families in the lives of youth.

Schools as a Source of Nonparent Adult Support

Teacher support has been consistently linked with higher levels of school engagement and performance, social competence, and self-esteem.[21] Children and adolescents spend a large proportion of their time in academic settings, so schools represent a natural and efficient site for facilitating the development of supportive adult-student relationships. Nonetheless, although schools are the site of nearly 75 percent of the preventive interventions for children and adolescents (for example, life skills training, smoking prevention),[22] such interventions tend to be somewhat short-term, disjointed efforts that are added onto classroom activities, rather than integrated into the schools' existing structures.[23] The supportive potential of teachers has not gone entirely unnoticed among school reformers, who recommend a broad array of efforts to directly capitalize on it. The influential Carnegie Council on Adolescent Development has called for schools to create "communities of learning, where stable, close, mutually respectful relationships with adults and peers are considered fundamental for intellectual development and personal growth."[24] Practices such as homeroom assignments, advising, multi-year teacher placements, and smaller groupings of students have been increasingly advocated in recent years.

Although these efforts have met with some success, close and confiding student-teacher relationships tend to be more the exception than the rule. Students may develop one or two important ties with certain teachers over the course of their schooling, but they do not perceive their typical teacher relationships as particularly close or meaningful.[25] Given the way schools are structured, this is not particularly surprising. The same teachers who are being asked to provide more personalized support are being saddled with additional obligations. A growing emphasis on high-stakes standardized testing has given rise to dense curricular demands that have constrained teachers and left little room for the sorts of conversations and activities that typically draw them closer to their students. Larger student/teacher ratios have left each young person with a smaller piece of the teacher's attention.

Sadly, many adults who were initially drawn to the teaching profession out of desire to establish meaningful connections with their students have become increasingly disillusioned by the structural impediments to relationships in schools. Supportive bonds become even less practical as students move into middle and high school and no longer have a primary teacher with whom they spend most of the day. Researchers have noted that middle school students tend to have few positive interactions outside of instruction and feel less secure with their teachers than do elementary school students.[26]

Although these changes may be due in part to normal developmental changes, such as increased orientation to peers and needs for independence, the less voluntary aspects of this loss of adult support are cause for concern. Relationships with certain teachers sometimes take on great importance during adolescence. Rather than presenting impediments, schools should increase the likelihood of such occurrences. As Jeannie Oakes and her colleagues concluded, "Students and schools cannot thrive if care is confined to private, occasional moments: a teacher, a principal who stops because she notices a child in tears; a coach available after school; a friend who will listen at lunch."[27]

A major challenge for schools will be to create settings that can increase and facilitate teachers' and other staff's caring potential, while maintaining academic rigor and teacher autonomy. Along these lines, school policies should be viewed in terms of how they may constrain or facilitate positive adult-student relationships.

In addition to making teacher salaries more competitive (the starting salaries of New York city teachers hover around $30,000 per year) and establishing a corps of highly qualified and high-quality teachers, we should evaluate school policies in terms of their effects on student-adult relationships. There is unequivocal evidence that lowered student-teacher ratios are associated with improved student achievement and competence, and this is a straightforward means of improving teacher-student interactions.[28] Similarly, policies that ensure more contact and continuity with teachers, such as homerooms and multi-year teacher assignments, might provide students with "the opportunity to learn one relationship, learn it well, and glean the developmental benefits of learning it."[29] This will involve moving beyond the typical piecemeal approach to service delivery in schools, characterized by Pianta and Walsh as, "pullout, add-on, short-term programs that are conducted by someone other than the classroom teacher."

Youth Development Programs

Adolescents' needs for attention and supervision do not end when the last bell of the day rings. A growing number of children are enrolled in school- and community-based after-school programs that promote learning, protect youth from negative peer pressure, and create opportunities for them to form relationships with caring, nonparent adults. Funds are flowing from public and private sectors to create and strengthen these after-school programs. For example, in 1998, the U.S. Department of Education launched the Twenty-First Century Community Learning Center program by awarding support to rural and inner-city schools to create safe, drug-free supervised environments for children and youth during non-school hours.

Community-based youth organizations such as Boy Scouts and Girl Scouts, YMCA, and Boys' and Girls' Clubs of America are important contexts for positive youth development. Such programs have been shown to provide youth with a sense of safety, adult guidance, and opportunities to take initiative and engage in socially desirable activities.[30] Researchers have characterized such contexts as bridges between the streets and mainstream culture.[31] As Michelle Fine and Lois Weis observed, they are spaces "in which people, potentially across all ages, come together to critique what is, shelter themselves from what has been, redesign what might be, and/or imagine what could be."[32] Since many of the adults who gather or work in such settings are from the same community that they serve, they are well positioned to be natural mentors for adolescents.[33]

Bart Hirsch and his colleagues recently examined adolescents' relationships with adult staff in several Boys' and Girls' Clubs.[34] Particularly for older adolescents, club staff were found to offer a distinct form of support, falling somewhere between the caring and love received from extended family and the more specific targeted skills received from adults at school. The majority of youth attended the club every day, and three-quarters of adolescents considered the club "a second home." Moreover, staff support was strongly related to adolescents' sense of well-being.

School and community-based after-school programs are unevenly distributed across and within communities.[35] After-school programs for low-income youth tend to be poorly funded, with most of the new funding going to a narrow band of programs.[36] And since no uniform standards or regulations apply to after-school programs across the country, wide variation in ratios and staff qualifications can be found.

These organizational limitations constrain youth's experiences in predictable ways. For example, although a wide variety of activities and more flexible programming tend to give rise to more positive staff-child interactions, programs in low-income neighborhoods often lack the sufficient resources to achieve these goals.[37] They offer relatively few extracurricular sports and activities and are often funded to address specific risks and problems. Similarly, although fewer students per staff give rise to warmer, more sensitive and supportive interactions, ratios in many programs hover around 25:1. Given their potential benefits to youth, a greater investment in such programs should be a priority among policy makers.

Despite widespread enthusiasm and burgeoning interest among college students in volunteerism, community-based programs are likely to remain hobbled by their inability to attract a steady flow of committed staff. Without adequate salary incentives for teaching and youth service jobs, the cadres of young adults who are inspired by their volunteer service experiences will be drawn away from a more sustained commitment to the needs of youth. In addition to attracting, certifying, and retaining staff, adequate, long-term investments are needed to establish an infrastructure of facilities and supports to uphold the quality of these programs in future years.

Program investment need not emerge only within the public sector. "Social entrepreneurs" who apply venture capital to social problems are becoming an important force in youth development initiatives. Organizations such as Teach for America, which draws college graduates into two-year teaching commitments in low-income urban and rural communities, or City Year, an urban equivalent of the Peace Corps, are stimulating new practices and ideas that could be brought to scale with government assistance. Additionally, recent collaborations between public and private initiatives, such as the government's AmeriCorps joining forces with the private America's Promise, are likely to lead to interesting, sustained programming for youth.

Also promising are State Mentoring Partnerships (such as the California Mentor Initiative, the Massachusetts Mentoring Partnership, the Minnesota Mentoring Partnership), which are collaboratively funded through public and private sources and are active in seventeen states. The government can extend its funds through the private investments and the services of volunteers, and the private sector benefits from government structure and financing.

Outreach and Services

Other settings can also be a rich source of adult support and guidance for youth. Religious communities often provide ongoing encouragement and mentoring through youth outreach and services. Gary Walker and Marc Freedman have argued that since social policies in general, and mentoring programs in particular, often do not reach or support the most severely disadvantaged youth, churches often play a critical support role.[38] This is particularly true in urban, black churches, which tend to be socially active in their communities and participate in a wide range of community programs.[39] Religious involvement is associated with lower delinquency among young people and plays an important role in the after-school lives of urban youth.[40]

Sipe and Ma tracked the discretionary time of adolescents in three cities and found that, along with positive youth development programs, churches and church-based programs were significant protective factors in the lives of urban youth.[41] As John DiIulio recently concluded, "Where secular mentoring and conventional social services programs for poor urban youth typically end, churches and religious outreach ministries often begin."[42] Since religious communities can be a source of strength to many adolescents, partnerships aimed at supporting the development of youth are warranted. Along these lines, the federal government has increasingly advocated for faith-based mentoring programs for children of parents who are in prison. Leading such efforts is the Philadelphia Church

Mentoring Network, which encompasses nearly 70 churches who work together to recruit, train, and support mentors for more than 700 urban youth.[43]

Vulnerable youth often come in contact with publicly funded service systems, such as welfare, juvenile justice, housing, and teen-parenting programs. Adolescents entering these systems are less likely than others to gain access to mentoring or other youth development programs. Although many such youth would benefit from the support of adults, these systems rarely capitalize on this caring potential. The programs are often inaccessible, disconnected from each other, and staffed with professionals who are burdened with large caseloads. With more deliberate planning, such settings could be made more responsive to the needs of youth.

Conclusions and Recommendations

Meaningful relationships between adults and adolescents can occur in many contexts, ranging from highly structured, arranged relationships to the more spontaneous yet influential ties that sometimes arise with cherished aunts and uncles, teachers, or clergy. Although my focus has been on volunteer relationships, adolescents encounter caring adults in many other contexts. Indeed, as I wrote this book, I was moved by the many stories that students, colleagues, and friends shared about the important adults who had taken them under their wings. It is clear that, even in a culture characterized by overwork, class divisions, and a lack of civic involvement, meaningful ties between natural mentors and adolescents can and do flourish.

Although it is tempting to argue for a more caring society that would render contrived mentoring relationships unnecessary, it is a mistake to be anything less than vigilant in supporting a full array of resources for caring relationships with adults. Changes in families, work demands, and communities have left many adolescents bereft of the adult supports that were available just a few decades ago, while presenting them with increasingly complex challenges. No one institution—whether families, schools, church, or after-school programs—can completely compensate for the social isolation that many children and adolescents experience, and each institution is stretched by the limitations of the others. Different youth derive benefits from different resources, and mentoring and other youth programs can protect them against negative choices and support their healthy development.

Fortunately, the economic growth of the 1990s, the rise in charitable donations, the spread of social entrepreneurship, a public willingness to spend more on family-friendly policies, education and after-school programs, and corporate involvement and investment in mentoring and other youth development programs, have created powerful opportunities for catch-up.

Funding Issues

Higher levels of public spending for mentoring programs are not likely to be embraced with universal enthusiasm. When politicians embrace mentoring as a means of helping vulnerable youth, it is often because people construe it as an alternative to a comprehensive publicly funded response.

Mentoring and other youth development programs are a supplement, not an alternative to, systematic school reform, job opportunities, health coverage, childcare, affordable housing, neighborhood revitalization, and public safety. Asking mentoring, or any other intervention strategy, to compensate for an anemic public investment in youth is a recipe for disappointment.

Even when mentoring programs are placed in the proper context, many policy makers and interventionists are seduced by what appears to be a relatively low price tag associated with mentoring programs. A more detailed cost-benefit analysis might help demolish this myth and convince policy makers of both the costs of taking a haphazard approach and the benefits of generous, sustained investment in mentoring. Cost-effectiveness analyses, which combine cost data with outcome data, can provide a foundation for such efforts.[44]

For example, Douglas Fountain and Amy Arbreton determined that although there was considerable variation, the median cost of a one-on-one relationship was just over $1,000 per year, and that programs typically leverage volunteer time and donated goods and services that essentially match every dollar in the budget.[45] Programs like Big Brothers Big Sisters provide extensive support. They require a one-year commitment from volunteers, whom they recruit, screen, and counsel. To be effective, mentors must commit for the long haul; mentoring cannot be a half-hearted effort. And volunteers need support from the programs that recruit them. If the government wants to promote volunteer programs, it must act in the same way: it must offer more than mere praise for volunteers; it must also commit for the long haul, making sure these mentoring initiatives have the money they need to help their mentors succeed. An important challenge for evaluators will be to document relationships between higher expenditures and greater benefits.

Obviously there is no way to put a dollar estimate onto all of the problems that are prevented or all of the doors that are opened as a result of having or being a mentor. But even crude estimates can help shape policy debates. Such estimates would also help to situate mentoring on a continuum of intensity in youth programming. Intensity tends to imply higher costs, so another function of cost-benefit analysis will be to more precisely calibrate adolescents' needs with the necessary level and expense of the youth development program. Certain youth might be responsive only to highly structured, one-on-one relationships, while others are perfectly adept at eliciting support from adults in informal group contexts. Youth who would be most appropriately referred to mentoring programs are those who, by virtue of their stress-laden environments, shyness, or other factors, would not readily find mentors in their everyday lives. Matching such youth with supportive adults can have marked effects on their adjustment.

Without such calculations and precision, and in a climate of unrealistic expectations, there is a danger that mentoring will become yet another in the litany of programs that have circulated into and out of the limelight. Mentoring should be given a fair chance to perform. It could be argued that the success of many human services initiatives essentially comes down to the quality of relationships that are forged among participants. By putting relationships at center stage, mentoring can deliver this healing in full potency. But a good performance requires a concerted "behind the scenes" effort and a supporting cast that upholds each mentor-protégé match in all of its complexity.

In the absence of this support, mentoring programs could lose constituents before they achieve their full potential. And, since the public is relatively impatient for solutions, the stakes are high. Freedman noted that heightened expectation for relationships to thrive in the absence of support and realistic goals—that is, fervor without infrastructure—"is dangerous at the policy level because it plays into the unfortunate tendency to lunge at new and glossy strategies, glorify them over the short term, and discard them as they tarnish. More disturbing is the way that fervor without infrastructure feeds the recurring appetite for voluntaristic panaceas, idealized in isolation from institutions, and proposed as quick, cheap, and easy."[46]

Into the Future

The future of mentoring, as a popularly embraced strategy is not entirely clear, and its current popularity carries certain risks. The atmosphere of hyperbole and expectations has created a large constituency and rare opportunities for high-quality programming and evaluation. But it has also placed enormous pressure on mentoring as an intervention strategy. It is working against the clock.

Uneven quality and exaggerated claims has already generated a fair amount of cynicism. In the face of day-to-day problems and less than obvious short-term benefits, some service providers are growing dispirited and expressing skepticism about whether mentoring is all that it's cracked up to be. Complaints that volunteerism is "only a Band-Aid when what is really needed is systemic change" or that "mentoring is as chancy as a blind date—and no more likely to lead to the lasting and solid relationships these kids need" abound.[47] Others worry about the inherent contradictions of having volunteer mentors "parachuting" into children's lives. A cover story of the *New York Times Magazine* recently characterized mentoring as little more than a feel-good vanity for middle-class adults that distracts their attention from more entrenched social problems.[48]

Such discouraging conclusions should be analyzed and vigorously countered. It is a mistake to create a false dichotomy between volunteering and government-funded initiatives, since both are needed and each strengthens the other. It is also a mistake to minimize the potential benefits of enduring mentoring relationships. Few would argue that parents' or teachers' inability to directly redress societal problems diminishes their importance. On the contrary, their role in protecting young lives from problems that stem from inequality, racism, violence, and isolation, and providing a bridge into new possibilities, becomes ever more significant. Mentoring should not be construed as a substitute for a more equitable distribution of material resources or a concerted youth policy agenda.

Nor should we minimize the political implications of connecting middle-class voters with at-risk youth. Mentoring can provide a lens through which middle-class adults can see the ravages of poverty: decrepit schools with stressed teachers, unsafe neighborhoods, deteriorating housing, and other difficult circumstances. Although many of us already know that one in five of the children in this wealthy democracy live in poverty, this inequality is somehow compartmentalized and largely ignored. Deeply connecting with one child in poverty can illuminate its pernicious effects, and is likely to mobilize more sustained authentic action. Support for a coordinated, public response to the out-of-school needs of school-aged youth is more likely to emerge when mentors see how their protégés' problems multiply during unsupervised hours. Through this process, mentoring can develop new constituencies for youth programs and policy.

Of course, mentors are also inspired by the many sources of strength in low-income and minority neighborhoods. When middle-class mentors bear witness to the caring that occurs in families, churches, and grassroots community organizations, and the level of commitment that urban parents marshal in support of their children, negative stereotypes are challenged.

Mentoring can serve as a pathway out of the poverty that often extends across generations. As illustrated by Nancy and Angela in Chapter 1, when mentors encourage low-income youth to engage in school and learning and to complete their education, they are also helping youth to disrupt cycles of economic deprivation and stressful environments. Additionally, mentoring programs provide a context for college-aged volunteers to observe public service at work and to engage in a world that extends beyond the narrow confines of their nuclear families. Since early civic participation is the best predictor of lifelong commitment, mentoring can provide an important training ground for future volunteerism.[49]

Another beneficial byproduct of mentoring is its role in garnering support for other youth development initiatives. Mentoring is intuitively appealing and easy to grasp, and the familiar, well-regarded Big Brothers Big Sisters organization confers other less-known programs with credibility and public support. In this sense, successful mentoring plays a role as a gateway toward the public's expanding commitment to youth policies, programs, and institutions.[50] Thus, we should neither minimize mentors' benefits to youth nor ignore the political implications of connecting largely middle-class adults with at-risk youth.

Much remains to be done to understand the complexities of mentor relationships and to determine the circumstances under which mentoring programs make a difference in the lives of youth. At this stage, we can safely say that mentoring is, by and large, a modestly effective intervention for youth who are already coping relatively well under somewhat difficult circumstances. In some cases it can do more harm than good; in others it can have extraordinarily influential effects. The balance can, and should, be tipped toward the latter. A deeper understanding of nonparent adult relationships, combined with high quality programs and enriched settings, will better position us to harness the full potential of youth mentoring.

Notes

Acknowledgments

Index

Notes

Names of volunteers, staff, and protégés have been changed to protect the privacy of individuals.

Introduction

1. C. L. Sipe and A. E. Roder, *Mentoring School-Age Children: A Classification of Programs* (Philadelphia: Public/Private Ventures; Arlington, VA: The National Mentoring Partnership, 1999). This publication, which was prepared for the National Mentoring Partnership's Public Policy Council, codifies the various approaches to mentoring.

2. J. B. Grossman and J. P. Tierney, "Does mentoring work? An impact study of the Big Brothers/Big Sisters," *Evaluation Review* 22 (1998): 403–426.

3. I have kept the technical details about statistics and research design to a minimum. Readers who are interested in the scientific reports from my ten years of work on mentoring are referred to the professional journals cited throughout this book.

4. J. E. Rhodes, "Mentoring programs," in A. E. Kazdin, ed., *Encyclopedia of Psychology* (Washington, DC: American Psychological Association, 2000).

5. Sipe and Roder, *Mentoring School-Age Children.*

1. Inventing a Promising Future

1. P. L. Benson, N. Leffert, P. C. Scales, and D. Blyth, "Beyond the 'village' rhetoric: Creating healthy communities for children and adolescents," *Applied Developmental Science* 2 (1998): 138–159.

2. T. M. Williams and W. Kornblum, *Growing Up Poor* (Lexington, MA: Lexington Books, 1985), p. 108.

3. B. Lefkowitz, *Tough Change: Growing Up on Your Own in America* (New York: Free Press, 1986), p. 117.

4. L. M. Burton, "Age norms, the timing of family role transitions, and intergenerational caregiving among aging African American women," *Gerontologist* 36 (1996): 199–208.

5. P. H. Collins, "The meaning of motherhood in black culture and black mother/daughter relationships," *Sage: A Scholarly Journal in Black Women* 4 (1987): 3–10.

6. C. B. Stack, *All Our Kin* (New York: Harper and Row, 1974).

7. O. Ramirez, "Mexican American children and adolescents," in J. T. Gibbs and L. N. Huang, eds., *Children of Color: Psychological Interventions with Minority Youth* (San Francisco: Jossey-Bass, 1989).

8. G. Caplan, *Principles of Preventive Psychiatry* (New York: Basic Books, 1964), p. 49.

9. E. L. Cowen, "Help is where you find it: Four informal helping groups," *American Psychologist* 37(4) (1982): 385–395.

10. S. R. Beier, W. D. Rosenfeld, K. C. Spitalny, S. M. Zanksy, and A. N. Bontemmpo, "The potential role of an adult mentor in influencing high-risk behaviors in adolescents," *Archives of Pediatric Medicine* 154 (2000): 327–331.

11. M. A. Zimmerman, J. B. Bingenheimer, and P. C. Notaro, "Natural mentors and adolescent resiliency: A study with urban youth," *American Journal of Community Psychology* (in press).

12. J. E. Rhodes, P. L. Gingiss, and P. B. Smith, "Risk and protective factors for alcohol use among pregnant African American, Hispanic, and White adolescents: The influence of peers, sexual partners, family members, and mentors," *Addictive Behaviors* 19 (1994): 555–564; J. E. Rhodes and A. A. Davis, "Supportive ties between nonparent adults and urban adolescent girls," in B. J. Leadbeater and N. Way, eds., *Urban Girls: Resisting Stereotypes, Creating Identities* (New York: New York University Press, 1996), pp. 213–249; E. L. Klaw and J. E. Rhodes, "Mentor relationships and the career development of African-American pregnant and parenting adolescents," *Psychology of Women Quarterly* 19 (1995): 551–562; J. E. Rhodes, L. Ebert, and K. Fischer, "Natural mentors: An overlooked resource in the social networks of young, African-American mothers," *American Journal of Community Psychology* 20 (1992): 445–461; J. E. Rhodes, J. M. Contreras, and S. C. Mangelsdorf, "Natural mentor relationships among Latina adolescent mothers: Psychological adjustment, moderating processes, and the role of early parental acceptance," *American Journal of Community Psychology* 22 (1994): 211–228.

13. F. F. Furstenberg, "How families manage risk and opportunity in dangerous neighborhoods," in W. J. Wilson, ed., *Sociology and the Public Agenda* (Newbury Park, CA: Sage, 1994): 231–258; R. D. Putnam, *Bowling Alone: The Collapse and Revival of American Community* (New York: Simon & Schuster, 2000).

14. R. J. Sampson, "Family management and child development: Insights from social disorganization theory," in J. McCord, ed., *Facts, Frameworks, and Forecasts: Advances in Criminological Theory* (New Brunswick, NJ: Transaction Publishers, 1992), pp. 63–93; E. Anderson, *Code of the Street: Decency, Violence, and the Moral Life of the Inner City* (New York: Norton, 1999), p. 287.

15. Wilson, *When Work Disappears*.

16. P. C. Scales, P. L. Benson, and E. C. Roehlkepastain, *Grading Grown-Ups: American Adults Report on Their Real Relationships with Kids* (Minneapolis: Lutheran Brotherhood and Search Institute, 2001).

17. R. Dawes, *House of Cards: Psychology and Psychotherapy Built on Myth* (New York: Simon & Schuster, 1996).

18. J. McKnight, *The Careless Society: Community and Its Counterfeits* (New York: Basic Books, 1995), pp. ix–x; Benson, Leffert, Scales, and Blyth, "Beyond the 'village' rhetoric."

19. D. A. Kleiber, *Leisure Experiences and Human Development: A Dialectical Interpretation* (New York: Basic Books, 1999).

20. N. Darling, S. F. Hamilton, and K. Hames, "Relationships outside the family: unrelated adults," *Blackwell Encyclopedia of Adolescence* (in press).

21. D. Belle, *The After-School Lives of Children: Alone and with Others While Parents Work* (Mahwah, NJ: Lawrence Erlbaum, 1999).

22. L. D. Steinberg, *Adolescence* (New York: McGraw-Hill, 1999).

23. Ibid.

24. Carnegie Council on Adolescent Development, *Turning Points: Preparing American Youth for the Twenty-First Century* (New York: Carnegie Corporation, 1989).

25. M. Freedman, *The Kindness of Strangers: Adult Mentors, Urban Youth, and the New Volunteerism* (San Francisco: Jossey-Bass, 1993).

26. M. Katz, *In the Shadow of the Poorhouse: A Social History of Welfare in America* (New York: Basic Books, 1997).

27. G. Manza, personal communication.

28. Ibid.

29. Freedman, *The Kindness of Strangers*.

30. Putnam, *Bowling Alone*.

31. E. Seligson, "The policy climate for school-age child care," *The Future of children* 9(2) (1999): 145–159.

32. R. W. Larson, "Toward a psychology of positive youth development," *American Psychologist* 55 (2000): 170–183; K. Hein, "Priorities in the study of adolescent development," in R. Lerner, chair, *Developmental Assets and Asset-Building Communities: Implications for Research, Policy, and Practice* (Paper presented at the Annual Meeting of the American Psychological Association, Washington, DC, August, 2000); R. M. Lerner, "Developing civil society through the promotion of positive youth development," *Journal of Developmental and Behavioral Pediatrics* 21 (2000): 48–49.

33. J. Roth, J. Brooks-Gunn, L. Murray, and W. Foster, "Promoting healthy adolescents: Synthesis of youth development program evaluations," *Journal of Research on Adolescence* 8(4) (1998): 423–459.

34. P. L. Benson, *All Kids Are Our Kids: What Communities Must Do to Raise Caring and Responsible Children and Adolescents* (San Francisco: Jossey-Bass, 1997).

35. S. Zeldin and L. Price, eds., "Creating supportive communities for adolescent development: Challenges to scholars," *Journal of Adolescent Research* 10(1) (1995).

36. J. M. McPartland and S. M. Nettles, "Using community adults as advocates or mentors for at-risk middle school students: A two-year evaluation of project RAISE," *American Journal of Education* 99 (1991): 568–586; W. S. Davidson and R. Redner, "The prevention of juvenile delinquency: Diversion from the juvenile justice system," in R. H. Price, E. L. Cowen, R. P. Lorion, and J. Ramos-McKay, eds., *Fourteen Ounces of Prevention: Theory, Research, and Prevention* (New York: Pergamon, 1988), pp. 123–137; A. S. Taylor, L. LoSciuto, M. Fox, S. M. Hilbert, and M. Sonkowsky, "The mentoring factor: Evaluation of the across ages' intergenerational approach to drug abuse prevention," *Child and Youth Services* 20(1–2) (1999): 77–99; D. L. DuBois and H. A. Neville, "Youth mentoring: Investigation of relationship characteristics and perceived benefits," *Journal of Community Psychology* 25 (1997): 227–234; G. Cave and J. Quint, *Career Beginnings Impact Evaluation: Findings from a Program for Disadvantaged High School Students* (New York: Manpower Demonstrations Research Corporation, 1990).

37. See J. B. Grossman and J. P. Tierney, "Does mentoring work? An impact study of the Big Brothers/Big Sisters," *Evaluation Review* 22 (1998): 403–426, for additional information.

38. The following instruments were administered: The Inventory of Parent and Peer Attachment (IPPA; G. S. Armsden and M. T. Greenberg, "Inventory of parent and peer attachment: Individual differences in their relationship to psychological well-being in adolescence," *Journal of Youth and Adolescence* 16 [1987]: 427–453); Features of

Children's Friendship Scale (T. Berndt and B. Perry, "Children's perceptions of friendships as supportive relationships," *Developmental Psychology* 22 [1986]: 640–648); the Inventory of School Value (T. Berndt and K. Miller, "Expectancies, values, and achievement in junior high school," *Journal of Educational Psychology* 82 [1986]: 319–326); Self-Perception Profile for Children (S. Harter, "The self-perception profile for children," University of Denver [1986]; Inventory of School Value (T. Berndt and K. Miller "Expectancies, values, and achievement in junior high school," *Journal of Educational Psychology* 82 [1986]: 319–326); and the Mentor Scale (M. B. Styles and K. V. Morrow, *Understanding How Youth and Elders Form Relationships: A Study of Four "Linking Lifetimes" Programs* [Philadelphia: Public/Private Ventures, 1992]). In addition, individual questions regarding the adolescents' background, functioning, and mentoring relationship were administered to the adolescents, their parents, and caseworkers.

39. Agency staff reported three major reasons for the failure to match the 109 treatment youth during the study period. Thirty-three of them became ineligible because the parent remarried, the youth was no longer within the eligible age range, or the youth's place of residence changed. Thirty-one were not matched because the youth no longer wanted a Big Brother or Big Sister. Twenty-one were not matched because a suitable volunteer could not be found during the study period. The 24 remaining treatment youth were not matched for a variety of reasons, most commonly because the parent or youth did not follow through with the intake process. To avoid biases in the measurement of mentoring effects, both matched and unmatched treatment participants were included in the analyses.

40. Grossman and Tierney, "Does mentoring work?"

41. J. Cohen, *Statistical Power Analysis for the Behavioral Sciences*, 2nd ed. (Hillsdale, NJ: Lawrence Erlbaum, 1988); Mark Lipsey, *Design Sensitivity: Statistical Power for Experimental Research* (Newbury Park, CA: Sage Publications, 1990), pp. 51–56. Computing effect sizes in program evaluations typically involves calculating the standardized differences between two means (called d-Family statistics). McCartney and Rosenthal point out that, in practice, researchers rarely obtain d's as large as .80 and, when these conventions are applied blindly, meaningful results can sometimes be mistakenly dismissed as trivial.

42. D. L. DuBois, B. E. Holloway, H. Cooper, and J. C. Valentine, "Effectiveness of mentoring programs for youth: A meta-analytic review," *American Journal of Community Psychology* (in press): 34.

43. Steinberg, *Adolescence*.

44. J. B. Grossman and J. E. Rhodes, "The test of time: Predictors and

effects of duration in youth mentoring programs," *American Journal of Community Psychology* (in press).

45. DuBois et al. (in press).

46. Ibid.

47. J. A. Durlak and A. M. Wells, "Primary prevention mental health programs for children and adolescents: A meta-analytic review," *American Journal of Community Psychology* 25(2) (April 1997): 115–152; M. W. Lipsey, and D. B. Wilson, "The efficacy of psychological, educational, and behavioral treatment: Confirmation from meta-analysis," *American Psychologist* 48(12) (December 1993): 1181–1209; J. Hattie, H. W. Marsh, J. T. Neill, and G. E. Richards, "Adventure education and outward bound: Out-of-class experiences that make a lasting difference," *Review of Educational Research* 67(1) (Spring 1997): 43–87.

48. C. Herrera, C. L. Sipe, W. S. McClanahan, with A. J. Arbreton and S. K. Pepper, *Mentoring School-Age Children: Relationship Development in Community-Based and School-Based Programs* (Philadelphia: Public/Private Ventures; Arlington, VA: The National Mentoring Partnership, 2000).

49. C. L. Sipe, "Mentoring adolescents: What have we learned," in J. B. Grossman, ed., *Contemporary Issues in Mentoring* (Philadelphia: Public/Private Ventures, 1998).

2. How Successful Mentoring Works

1. R. J. Haggerty, L. R. Sherrod, N. Garmezy, and M. Rutter, eds., *Stress, Risk, and Resilience in Children and Adolescents: Processes, Mechanisms, and Interventions* (New York: Cambridge University Press, 1996).

2. A. S. Masten and J. D. Coatsworth, "The development of competence in favorable and unfavorable environments: Lessons from research on successful children," *American Psychologist* 53(2) (February 1998): 205–220.

3. N. Garmezy, "Stress resistant children: The search for protective Factors," in J. E. Stevenson, ed., *Recent Research in Developmental Psychopathology* (Oxford: Pergamon, 1985), p. 227.

4. F. F. Furstenburg, T. D. Cook, J. Eccles, G. H. Elder, and A. Sameroff, *Managing to Make It: Urban Families and Adolescent Success* (Chicago: University of Chicago Press, 1999).

5. N. Darling, S. Hamilton, T. Toyokawa, and S. Matsuda, "Naturally-occurring mentoring in Japan and the United States: Social roles and correlates," *American Journal of Community Psychology* (in press).

6. Garmezy, "Stress resistant children."

7. Ibid., p. 227.

8. M. Rutter, "Protective factors in children's responses to stress and disadvantage," in M. W. Kent and J. E. Rolf, eds., *Primary Prevention of Psychopathology: Social Competence in Children* (Hanover, NH: University Press of New England, 1979), pp. 49–74; M. Rutter, "Psychosocial resilience and protective mechanisms," *American Journal of Orthopsychiatry* 57 (1987): 57–72.

9. M. Rutter and H. Giller, *Juvenile Delinquency: Trends and Perspectives* (New York: Guilford Press, 1983), p. 237.

10. E. E. Werner and R. S. Smith, *Vulnerable but Invincible: A Study of Resilient Children* (New York: McGraw-Hill, 1982).

11. See Masten and Coatsworth, "The development of competence in favorable and unfavorable environments."

12. S. S. Luthar and D. Cicchetti, "The construct of resilience: Implications for interventions and social policies," *Development and Psychopathology* 12 (2000): 857–885.

13. Ibid.

14. S. S. Luthar, "Vulnerability and resilience: A study of high-risk adolescents," *Child Development* 62(3) (1991): 600–616.

15. Werner and Smith, *Vulnerable but Invincible*.

16. M. E. Kenny and K. G. Rice, "Attachment to parents and adjustment in late adolescent college students: Current status, applications, and future considerations," *Counseling Psychologist* 23(3) (1995): 433–456.

17. M. Lynch and D. Cicchetti, "Children's relationships with adults and peers: An examination of elementary and junior high school students," *Journal of School Psychology* 35 (1997): 81–100.

18. E. Debold, L. M. Brown, S. Weseen, and G. K. Brookins, "Cultivating hardiness zones for adolescent girls: A reconceptualization of resilience in relationships with caring adults," in N. G. Johnson and M. C. Roberts, eds., *Beyond Appearance: A New Look at Adolescent Girls* (Washington, DC: American Psychological Association, 1999), pp. 181–204.

19. C. R. Cooper, H. D. Grotevant, and S. M. Condon, "Individuality and connectedness both foster adolescent identity formation and role taking skills," in H. D. Grotevant and C. R. Cooper, eds., *Adolescent Development in the Family*, New Directions for Child Development, 22 (San Francisco: Jossey-Bass, 1983), pp. 43–59.

20. M. A. Zimmerman, J. B. Bingenheimer, and P. C. Notaro, "Natural mentors and adolescent resiliency: A study with urban youth," *American Journal of Community Psychology* (in press); S. T. Hauser, S. I. Powers, and G. G. Noam, *Adolescents and Their Families: Paths of Ego Development* (New York: Free Press, 1991); N. Darling, S. F. Hamilton, and S. Niego, "Adolescents' relations with adults outside the family," in R. Monemayor

and G. R. Adams, eds., *Personal Relationships during Adolescence: Advances in Adolescent Development*, Annual Book Series, 6 (Thousand Oaks, CA: Sage Publications, 1994): 216–235; J. E. Rhodes, J. M. Contreras, and S. C. Mangelsdorf, "Natural mentor relationships among Latina adolescent mothers: Psychological adjustment, moderating processes, and the role of early parental acceptance," *American Journal of Community Psychology* 22 (1994): 211–228.

21. F. F. Furstenburg, T. D. Cook, J. Eccles, G. H. Elder, and A. Sameroff, *Managing to Make It: Urban Families and Adolescent Success* (Chicago: University of Chicago Press, 1999).

22. R. L. Jarrett, "Successful parenting in high-risk neighborhoods," *The Future of children* 9(2) (1999): 45–50.

23. W. A. Collins, and C. Luebker, "Parent and adolescent expectancies: Individual and relational significance," in J. G. Smetana, ed., *Beliefs about Parenting: Origins and Developmental Implications*, New Directions for Child Development, 66 (San Francisco: Jossey-Bass, 1994).

24. L. Steinberg, *Beyond the Classroom: Why School Reform Has Failed and What Parents Need to Do* (New York: Simon & Schuster, 1996); J. S. Eccles, "The development of children ages 6 to 14," *Future of Children* 9(2) (Fall 1999): 39.

25. Niobe Way, *Everyday Courage: The Lives and Stories of Urban Teenagers* (New York: New York University Press, 1998); D. J. Levinson, *The Seasons of a Man's Life* (New York: Ballantine Books, 1978).

26. R. W. Larson, "Toward a psychology of positive youth development," *American Psychologist* 55 (2000): 170–183.

27. C. Herrera, L. Sipe, and W. S. McClanahan, *Mentoring School-Age Children: Relationship Development in Community-Based and School-Based Programs* (Philadelphia: Public/Private Ventures, 2000); J. B. Grossman and J. E. Rhodes, "The test of time: Predictors and effects of duration in youth mentoring programs," *American Journal of Community Psychology* (in press).

28. S. F. Hamilton, and L. Darling, "Mentors in adolescents' lives," in Hurrelmann and U. Engel, eds., *The Social World of Adolescents* (New York: Walter de Gruyter, 1989).

29. Herrera, Sipe, and McClanahan, *Mentoring School-Age Children.*

30. H. Kohut, "The psychoanalyst in the community of scholars," in P. Ornstein, ed., *The Search for the Self: Selected Writings of Heinz Kohut* (New York: International Universities Press, 1978), pp. 685–724; D. W. Winnicott, *Playing and Reality* (New York: Basic Books, 1971); R. Schafer, "Generative empathy in the treatment situation," *Psychoanalytic Quarterly* 28(3) (1959): 342–373.

31. Kohut, "The psychoanalyst in the community of scholars," pp. 704–705; L. Delpit, *Other People's Children: Cultural Conflict in the Classroom* (New York: New York Press, 1995), p. 46.

32. J. V. Jordan, "The meaning of mutuality," in J. V. Jordan, A. G. Kaplan, J. B. Miller, I. P. Stiver, and J. L. Surrey, *Women's Growth in Connection: Writings from the Stone Center* (New York: Guilford Press, 1991).

33. M. B. Styles and K. V. Morrow, *Understanding How Youth and Elders Form Relationships: A Study of Four Linking Lifetimes Programs* (Philadelphia: Public/Private Ventures, 1995).

34. Jordan, "The meaning of mutuality."

35. H. Kohut, *How Does Analysis Cure?* (Chicago: University of Chicago Press: 1984), p. 78.

36. J. B. Grossman and J. P. Tierney, "Does mentoring work? An impact study of the Big Brothers/Big Sisters," *Evaluation Review* 22 (1998): 403–426. S. F. Hamilton and N. Darling, "Mentors in adolescents' lives," in K. Hurrelmann and S. F. Hamilton, eds., *Social Problems and Social Contexts in Adolescence: Perspectives across Boundaries* (New York: Aldine De Gruyter, 1996), pp. 199–215; J. E. Rhodes, J. M. Contreras, and S. C. Mangelsdorf, "Natural mentor relationships among Latina adolescent mothers: Psychological adjustment, moderating processes, and the role of early parental acceptance," *American Journal of Community Psychology* 22 (1994): 211–228.

37. Styles and Morrow, *Understanding How Youth and Elders Form Relationships.*

38. J. Bowlby, "Attachment and loss: Retrospect and prospect," *American Journal of Orthopsychiatry* 52 (1982): 664–676.

39. M. Ainsworth, "Attachments beyond infancy," *American Psychologist* 44 (1989): 709–716.

40. M. Lynch and D. Cicchetti, "Maltreated children's reports of relatedness to their teachers," in R. C. Pianta, ed., *Beyond the Parent: The Role of Other Adults in Children's Lives,* New Directions for Child Development, 57 (San Francisco: Jossey-Bass, 1992), p. 81.

41. L. A. Sroufe, E. A. Carlson, A. K. Levy, and B. Egeland, "Implications of attachment theory for developmental psychopathology," *Development and Psychopathology* 11(1) (Winter 1999): 1–13.

42. J. P. Allen and D. Land, "Attachment in adolescence," in J. Cassidy, P. R. Shaver, et al., eds., *Handbook of Attachment: Theory, Research, and Clinical Applications* (New York: Guilford Press, 1999), pp. 319–335. M. Main, N. Kaplan, and J. Cassidy, "Security in infancy, childhood, and adulthood: A move to the level of representation," in I. Bretherton and E. Waters, eds., *Growing Points of Attachment: Theory and Research,* Mono-

graphs of the Society for Research in Child Development, 209 (Philadelphia, 1985), pp. 3–35.

43. Allen and Land, "Attachment in adolescence."

44. R. C. Pianta, *Enhancing Relationships between Children and Teachers* (Washington, DC: American Psychological Association, 1999).

45. J. E. Rhodes, J. B. Grossman, and N. R. Resch, "Agents of change: Pathways through which mentoring relationships influence adolescents' academic adjustment," *Child Development* 91 (2000): 1662–1671.

46. C. H. Cooley, *Human Nature and the Social Order* (New York: Scribner, 1902).

47. G. H. Mead, *Mind, Self, and Society from the Standpoint of a Social Behaviorist* (Chicago: University of Chicago Press, 1934); H. Blumer, *Symbolic Interactionism: Perspective and Method* (Berkeley: University of California Press, 1980).

48. J. Bolby, *The Making and Breaking of Affectional Bonds* (London: Tavistock, 1979), p. 103.

49. D. P. Keating, "Adolescent thinking," in S. S. Feldman and G. R. Elliott, eds., *At the Threshold: The Developing Adolescent* (Cambridge: Harvard University Press, 1990).

50. B. Rogoff, *Apprenticeship in Thinking* (New York: Oxford University Press, 1990).

51. L. S. Vygotsky, *Mind in Society* (Cambridge: Harvard University Press, 1978).

52. B. Rogoff, *Apprenticeship in Thinking: Cognitive Development in Social Context* (New York: Oxford University Press, 1990); J. Wertsch, G. D. McNamee, J. B. McLane, and N. A. Budwig. "The adult-child dyad as a problem-solving system," in P. Llyod and C. Fernyhough, eds., *Lev Vygotsky: Critical Assessments: The Zone of Proximal Development*, vol. 3 (New York: Routledge. 1999).

53. L. M. Brown and C. Gilligan, *Meeting at the Crossroads: Women's Psychology and Girls' Development* (Cambridge: Harvard University Press, 1992).

54. N. Darling, S. F. Hamilton, and K. Hames, "Relationships outside the Family: Unrelated adults," *Blackwell Encyclopedia of Adolescence* (in press).

55. D. P. Keating, "Adolescent thinking," in Feldman and Elliott, eds., *At the Threshold*, p. 58.

56. R. W. Roeser, J. S. Eccles, and A. J. Sameroff, "Academic and emotional functioning in early adolescence: Longitudinal relations, patterns, and prediction by experience in middle school," *Development and Psychopathology* 10(2) (1998): 321–352; R. M. Ryan, J. D. Stiller, and J. H.

Lynch, "Representations of relationships to teachers, parents, and friends as predictors of academic motivation and self-esteem," *Journal of Early Adolescence* 14 (1994): 226–249.

57. Pianta, *Enhancing Relationships between Children and Teachers.*

58. E. A. Blechman, "Mentors for high-risk minority youth: From effective communication to bicultural competence," *Journal of Clinical Child Psychology* 21(2) (1992): 160–169.

59. Larson, "Toward a psychology of positive youth development."

60. T. Kemper, "Reference groups, socialization, and achievement," *American Sociological Review* 33 (1968): 31–45; A. Bandura, "Social learning theory of identification processes," in D. A. Goslin, ed., *Handbook of Socialization Theory and Research* (Chicago: Rand-McNally, 1969).

61. S. Freud, "On narcissism: An introduction," in J. Strachey, ed., *Standard Edition of the Complete Psychological Works of Sigmund Freud*, vol. 14 (1914), pp. 73–102.

62. Kohut, *How Does Analysis Cure?*

63. R. D. Putnam, *Bowling Alone: The Collapse and Revival of American Community* (New York: Simon & Shuster, 2000).

64. Darling et al., "Adolescents' relations with adults outside the family."

65. M. R. Beam, C. Chen, and E. Greenberger, "The nature of adolescents' relationships with their 'very important' non-parental Adults," *American Journal of Community Psychology* (in press); M. A. Zimmerman, J. B. Bingenheimer, and P. C. Notaro, "Natural mentors and adolescent resiliency: A study with urban youth," *American Journal of Community Psychology* (in press).

66. H. Markus, and P. Nurius, "Possible selves," *American Psychologist* 41(9) (September 1986): 954–969.

67. Levinson, *Seasons of a Man's Life.*

68. S. Harter, "Symbolic interactionism revisited: Potential liabilities for the self constructed in the crucible of interpersonal relationships," *Merrill-Palmer Quarterly* 45(4) (October 1999): 677–703.

69. S. Fordham and J. U. Ogbu, "Black students' school success: Coping with the 'burden of acting white,'" *Urban Review* 18(3) (1986): 176–206.

70. E. Debold, L. M. Brown, S. Weseen, and G. K. Brookins, "Cultivating hardiness zones for adolescent girls: A reconceptualization of resilience in relationships with caring adults," in N. G. Johnson and M. C. Roberts, eds., *Beyond Appearance: A New Look at Adolescent Girls* (Washington, DC: American Psychological Association, 1999), p. 47.

71. S. Harter, "Symbolic interactionism revisited: Potential liabilities

for the self constructed in the crucible of interpersonal relationships," *Merrill-Palmer Quarterly* 45(4) (1999): 677–703.

72. J. G. Roffman, C. Suarez-Orozco, and J. E. Rhodes, "Facilitating positive development in immigrant youth: The role of mentors and community organizers," in D. F. Perkins, L. M. Borden, J. G. Keith, and F. A. Villarrurel, eds., *Positive Youth Development: Creating a Positive Tomorrow* (New York: Klewer Press, in press).

73. N. Darling, S. Hamilton, T. Toyokawa, and S. Matsuda, "Naturally-occurring mentoring in Japan and the United States: Social roles and correlates," *American Journal of Community Psychology* (in press).

74. J. E. Rhodes, R. Reddy, and L. N. Osborne, "Protégé baseline characteristics as predictors of youth outcomes in mentoring programs" (unpub. ms, 2000).

75. J. W. Thibaut and H. H. Kelley, *The Social Psychology of Groups* (New Brunswick, NJ: Transaction Publishers, 1959).

76. F. Riessman, "The "helper-therapy" principle," *Social Work* 10(2) (1965): 27–32.

77. A. Taylor and J. Bressler, *Mentoring across Generations: Partnerships for Positive Youth Development* (New York: Kluwer Academic/Plenum Press, in press).

78. J. Armstrong, "I got it: Mentoring isn't for the mentor," *Newsweek* (June 2000): 87.

79. J. Katz, *Geeks: How Two Lost Boys Rode the Internet Out of Idaho* (New York: Random House, 2000).

80. E. H. Erikson, *Identity and the Life Cycle* (New York: W. W. Norton, 1994).

81. S. F. Schulz, "The benefits of mentoring," in M. W. Galbraith and N. H. Cohen, eds. *Mentoring: New strategies and Challenges*, New Directions for Adult and Continuing Education, 66 (San Francisco: Jossey-Bass, 1995).

82. M. Freedman, *Prime Time: How the Baby-Boomers Will Revolutionize Retirement and Transform America* (Washington, DC: Public Affairs, 1999).

83. S. G. Weinberger, *Allstate Mentoring Program* (Norfolk, CT: Mentoring Consulting Group, 2000).

84. C. Rosenberger, "Beyond empathy: Developing critical consciousness through service learning," in C. R. O'Grady, ed., *Integrating Service Learning and Multicultural Education in College and Universities* (Mahwah, NJ: Lawrence Erlbaum Associates, 2000); D. A. Blyth, R. Saito, and T. Berkas, "A quantitative study of the impact of service-learning programs," in A. S. Waterman et al., eds., *Service-Learning: Applications*

from the Research (Mahwah, NJ: Lawrence Erlbaum Associates, 1997), pp. 39–56.

3. The Risks of Relationships

1. M. Freedman, *The Kindness of Strangers: Adult Mentors, Urban Youth, and the New Volunteerism* (San Francisco: Jossey-Bass, 1993).

2. F. F. Furstenberg and A. J. Cherlin, *Divided Families: What Happens to Children When Parents Part* (Cambridge: Harvard University Press, 1991).

3. C. L. Sipe, *Mentoring: A Synthesis of P/PV's Research: 1988–1995* (Philadelphia: Public/Private Ventures, 1996).

4. M. B. Styles and K. V. Morrow, *Understanding How Youth and Elders Form Relationships: A Study of Four Linking Lifetimes Programs* (Philadelphia: Public/Private Ventures, 1995).

5. A. M. Omoto and M. Snyder, "Sustained helping without obligation: Motivation, longevity of service, and perceived attitude change among AIDS volunteers," *Journal of Personality and Social Psychology* 68 (1995): 671–686.

6. J. W. Thibaut and H. H. Kelley, *The Social Psychology of Groups* (New Brunswick, NJ: Transaction Publishers, 1959).

7. J. S. Wallerstein, "Children of divorce: Stress and developmental tasks," in N. Garmezy and M. Rutter, eds., *Stress, Coping and Development in Children* (Baltimore: Johns Hopkins University Press, 1988), pp. 265–302.

8. M. Lynch and D. Cicchetti, "Maltreated children's reports of relatedness to their teachers," in R. C. Pianta, ed., *Beyond the Parent: The Role of Other Adults in Children's Lives,* New Directions in Child Development, 57 (1992): 81–108.

9. G. Downey and S. I. Feldman, "The implications of rejection sensitivity for intimate relationships," *Journal of Personality and Social Psychology* 70 (1996): 1327–1343; J. X. Bembry and C. Ericson, "Therapeutic termination with the early adolescent who has experienced multiple losses," *Child and Adolescent Social Work Journal* 16(3) (1999): 177–189.

10. R. G. Simmons, R. Burgeson, and M. J. Reef, "Cumulative change at entry to adolescence," in M. R. Gunnar and W. A. Collins, eds., *Development during the Transition to Adolescence,* Minnesota Symposia on Child Psychology, 21 (Hillsdale, NJ: Lawrence Erlbaum Associates, 1988), p. 137.

11. J. Youniss and J. Smollar, *Adolescent Relations with Mothers, Fathers, and Friends* (Chicago: University of Chicago Press, 1985).

12. G. Noam, "The psychology of belonging: Reformulating adolescent development," in A. H. Esman, L. T. Flaherty, et al., eds., *Adolescent Psychiatry: Development and Clinical Studies*, Annals of the American Society for Adolescent Psychiatry, 24 (Hillsdale, NJ: Analytic Press, 1999).

13. J. Bowlby, *The Making and Breaking of Affectional Bonds* (London: Tavistock, 1979).

14. Downey and Feldman, "The implications of rejection sensitivity for intimate relationships."

15. E. Powers, and H. Witmer, *An Experiment in the Prevention of Delinquency: The Cambridge-Somerville Youth Study* (1951; Montclair, NJ: Patterson Smith, 1972); J. McCord, "A thirty-year followup of treatment effects," *American Psychologist* 33 (1978): 284–289.

16. L. W. Sherman, D. Gottfredson, D. MacKenzie, J. Eck, P. Reuter, and S. Bushway, *Preventing Crime: What Works, What Doesn't, What's Promising*, Report to the United States Congress (Washington, DC: National Institute of Justice, 1999).

17. E. K. Slicker and D. J. Palmer, "Mentoring at-risk school students: Evaluation of a school based program," *School Counselor*, 40 (1993): 327–334.

18. C. L. Sipe and A. E. Roder, *Mentoring School-Age Children: A Classification of Programs* (Philadelphia: Public/Private Ventures, 2000).

19. D. J. Levinson, with C. N. Darrow, E. B. Klein, M. H. Levinson, B. McKee, *The Seasons of a Man's Life* (New York: Ballantine Books, 1978), p. 101.

20. C. L. Sipe and A. E. Roder, *Mentoring School-Age Children: A Classification of Programs* (Philadelphia: Public/Private Ventures, 1999).

21. C. Herrera, L. Sipe, and W. S. McClanahan, *Mentoring School-Age Children: Relationship Development in Community-Based and School-Based Programs* (Philadelphia: Public/Private Ventures, 2000).

22. Sipe and Roder, *Mentoring School-Age Children.*

23. Herrera, Sipe, and McClanahan, *Mentoring School-Age Children.*

24. D. L. DuBois, B. E. Holloway, H. Cooper, and J. C. Valentine, "Effectiveness of mentoring programs for youth: A meta-analytic review," *American Journal of Community Psychology* (in press).

25. Ibid.

26. J. Bowlby, "The growth of independence in the young child," *Royal Society of Health Journal* 77 (1956): 587–591.

27. Larry E. Beutler, "Manualizing flexibility: The training of eclectic therapists," *Journal of Clinical Psychology* 55(4) (1999): 399–404.

28. G. W. Albee, "The Boulder model's fatal flaw," *American Psychologist* 55(2) (2000): 247–248.

29. Bachelor and Horvath, "The therapeutic relationship," in M. A. Hubble, B. L. Duncan, et al., eds., *The Heart and Soul of Change: What Works in Therapy* (Washington, DC: American Psychological Association, 1999).

30. C. Spear, *The Common Relational Landscape: A Psychological and Cultural Inquiry into Vicious Cycles of Abandonment* (Ann Arbor, MI: UMI Disserataion Services, 1998).

31. J. Bowlby, *A Secure Base: Parent-Child Attachment and Healthy Human Development* (New York: Basic Books, 1988); E. Erikson, *Childhood and Society* (New York: Norton, 1993); L. Kohlberg, *The Philosophy of Moral Development* (San Fransisco: Harper and Row, 1981).

32. J. Greenberg, and S. Mitchell, *Object Relations in Psychoanalytic Theory* (Cambridge: Harvard University Press, 1983), p. 3.

33. Jean Baker Miller, for example, has argued that the goal of development "is not for the individuals to grow out of relationship, but to grow into them. As the relationship grows, so grows the individual." For example, Carol Gilligan, "Women's Psychological Development: Implications for Psychotherapy," in C. Gilligan, A. Rogers, and D. Tolman, eds., *Women, Girls, and Psychotherapy: Reframing Resistance* (Binghamton, NY: 1991), highlighted the importance of remaining in relationship with oneself and others. Nancy Chodorow, "Toward a Relational Individualism: The Mediation of Self through Psychoanalysis," in T. Heller, M. Sosna, D. Wellbery, eds., *Reconstructing Individualism: Autonomy, Individuality, and Self in Western Thought* (Palo Alto: Stanford University Press, 1986), pp. 111–123, described development as occurring in a "relational matrix." Jessica Benjamin, "Recognition and Destruction: An Outing of Intersubjectivity," *Psychoanalytic Psychology* 7 (1990): 33–47, emphasized the "mutual recognition and attunement" that occurs when two people are in connection with other. These and other theorists imply that relationship-based interventions have the potential to influence fundamental processes that are central to healthy development.

34. H. S. Sullivan, *Interpersonal Theory of Psychiatry* (New York: Norton, 1953), pp. 21–262.

35. Ibid.

36. Spear, *The Common Relational Landscape*.

37. Jean Baker Miller and Irene P. Stiver, "The Healing Connection: How Women Form Relationships in Therapy and in Life" (Boston: Beacon Press, 1997).

38. J. B. Miller, "Connections, Disconnections, and Violations." Work

in Progress, 52 (Wellesley, MA: Stone Center Working Paper Series, 1998).

39. Ibid.

4. *Going the Distance*

1. P. A. Roaf, J. P. Tierney, and D. E. I. Hunte, *Big Brothers/Big Sisters of America: A Study of Volunteer Recruitment and Screening* (Philadelphia: Public/Private Ventures, 1994).

2. Ibid.

3. C. L. Sipe and A. E. Roder, *Mentoring School-Age Children: A Classification of Programs* (Philadelphia: Public Private Ventures, 1999).

4. Roaf et al., *Big Brothers/Big Sisters of America.*

5. J. B. Grossman and A. Johnson, "Assessing the effectiveness of mentoring programs," in J. B. Grossman, ed., *Contemporary Issues in Mentoring* (Philadelphia: Public/Private Ventures 1998), pp. 25–47.

6. Personal conversation with Steve Suimmi, April 2000.

7. M. Rutter, "Psychosocial influences: Critiques, findings, and research needs," *Development and Psychopathology* 12 (2000): 375–405; D. L. DuBois, B. E. Holloway, H. Cooper and J. C. Valentine, "Effectiveness of mentoring programs for youth: A meta-analytic review," *American Journal of Community Psychology* (in press).

8. C. L. Sipe, "Mentoring adolescents: What have we learned," in J. B. Grossman, ed., *Contemporary Issues in Mentoring* (Philadelphia: Public/Private Ventures, 1998).

9. C. L. Sipe, *Mentoring: A Synthesis of P/PV's Research: 1988–1995* (Philadelphia: Public/Private Ventures, 1996).

10. Sipe, "Mentoring adolescents."

11. Sipe and Roder, *Mentoring School-Age Children.*

12. M. B. Styles and K. V. Morrow, *Linking Lifetimes: Understanding How Youth and Elders Form Relationships* (Phildelphia: Public/Private Ventures, 1992).

13. J. B. Grossman and S. Jaccobi, *Strengthening Mentoring Programs* (Philadelphia: Public/Private Ventures, 2000).

14. A. Taylor and J. Bressler, *Mentoring across Generations: Partnerships for Positive Youth Development* (New York: Kluwer Academic/Plenum Press, in press).

15. J. B. Grossman and J. E. Rhodes, "The test of time: Predictors and effects of duration in youth mentoring programs," *American Journal of Community Psychology* (in press). Relationship length coded as 0 for all controls and unmatched treatment participants. The four length-of-

match dummy variables were entered into a regression equation for each outcome. The equations were estimated over the full sample of treatment youth. Because we were interested in explaining the changes during the eighteen-month period, not the level of the outcomes, we controlled for baseline levels of variables. Other baseline characteristics were also included in the models to reduce the variance unrelated to mentoring.

16. M. Lynch and D. Cicchetti, "Maltreated children's reports of relatedness to their teachers," in R. C. Pianta, ed., *Beyond the Parent: The Role of Other Adults in Children's Lives*, New Directions in Child Development, 57 (1992): 81–108.

17. G. Downey and S. I. Feldman, "The implications of rejection sensitivity for intimate relationships," *Journal of Personality and Social Psychology* 70 (1996): 1327–1343.

18. J. E. Rhodes, W. L. Haight, and E. Briggs, "The influence of mentoring on the peer relationships of foster youth in relative and nonrelative care," *Journal of Research on Adolescence* 9 (1999): 185–201.

19. A. M. Omoto and M. Snyder, "Sustained helping without obligation: Motivation, longevity of service, and perceived attitude change among AIDS volunteers," *Journal of Personality and Social Psychology* 68 (1995): 671–686.

20. Taylor and Bressler, *Mentoring across Generations*.

21. M. Freedman, *Prime Time: How the Baby-Boomers Will Revolutionize Retirement and Transform America* (Washington, DC: Public Affairs, 1999).

22. A. S. Taylor, L. LoSciuto, M. Fox, S. M. Hilbert, and M. Sonkowsky, "The mentoring factor: Evaluation of the across ages' intergenerational approach to drug abuse prevention," *Child and Youth Services* 20(1–2) (1999): 77–99.

23. D. L. DuBois, B. E. Holloway, H. Cooper, and J. C. Valentine, "Effectiveness of mentoring programs for youth: A meta-analytic review," *American Journal of Community Psychology* (in press).

24. J. E. Rhodes, R. Reddy, and L. N. Osborne, *Protégé Baseline Characteristics as Predictors of Youth Outcomes in Mentoring Programs* (unpub. ms., 2001).

25. Grossman and Johnson, "Assessing the effectiveness of mentoring programs."

26. B. Liang, A. J. Tracy, C. A. Taylor, and L. M. Williams, "Mentoring college-age women: A relational approach," *American Journal of Community Psychology* (in press).

27. E. A. Ensher and S. E. Murphy, "Effects of race, gender, perceived similarity, and contact on mentor relationships," *Journal of Vocational Behavior* 50(3) (1997): 460–481.

28. S. T. Fiske and S. E. Taylor, *Social Cognition*, 2nd ed. (New York: McGraw-Hill Book Company, 1991).

29. A. Bachelor, "Clients' perception of the therapeutic alliance: A qualitative analysis," *Journal of Counseling Psychology* 42(3) (1995): 323–337.

30. C. Herrera, L. Sipe, and W. S. McClanahan, *Mentoring School-Age Children: Relationship Development in Community-Based and School-Based Programs* (Philadelphia: Public/Private Ventures, 2000).

31. Sipe and Roder, *Mentoring School-Age Children.*

32. J. Ward, *The Skin We're In* (New York: Free Press, 2000).

33. G. L. Cohen, C. M. Steele, L. D. Ross, "The mentor's dilemma: Providing critical feedback across the racial divide," *Personality and Social Psychology Bulletin* 25(10) (1999): 1302–1318.

34. J. U. Ogbu, *Mentoring Minority Youth: A Framework* (New York: Columbia University, Teachers College, Institute for Urban and Minority Education, 1990; available from ERIC Document Reproduction Service, no. ED 354 293).

35. K. P. Furano, P. A. Roaf, M. B. Styles, and A. Y. Branch, *Big Brothers/Big Sisters: A Study of Program Practices* (Philadelphia: Public/Private Ventures, 1993).

36. R. F. Ferguson, *The Case for Community Based Programs that Inform and Motivate Black Male Youth* (Washington, DC: The Urban Institute, 1990), p. 19.

37. K. V. Morrow and M. B. Styles, *Building Relationships with Youth in Program Settings: A Study of Big Brothers/Big Sisters* (Philadelphia: Public/Private Ventures, 1995).

38. Herrera, Sipe, and McClanahan, *Mentoring School-Age Children.*

39. E. A. Blechman, "Mentors for high-risk minority youth: From effective communication to bicultural competence," *Journal of Clinical Child Psychology* 21(2) (1992): 160–169.

40. E. Flaxman, C. Ascher, and C. Harringon, *Youth Mentoring: Programs and Practices* (New York: Columbia University Teachers College, 1998; available from the ERIC Clearinghouse on Urban Education, Institute for Urban Minority Education, Box 40, Teachers College, Columbia University, New York, NY 10027), p. 3.

41. M. R. Edelman, *Lanterns: A Memoir of Mentors* (Boston: Beacon Press, 1999).

42. J. E. Rhodes, R. Reddy, and J. B. Grossman (in press). "Volunteer mentoring relationships with minority youth: An analysis of same- versus cross-race matches," *Journal of Applied Social Psychology.*

43. Grossman and Johnson, "Assessing the effectiveness of mentoring programs."

44. Herrera, Sipe, and McClanahan, *Mentoring School-Age Children.*

45. Grossman and Johnson, "Assessing the effectiveness of mentoring programs"; D. L. DuBois and H. A. Neville, "Youth mentoring: Investigation of relationship characteristics and perceived benefits," *Journal of Community Psychology* 25 (1997): 227–234; Morrow and Styles, *Building Relationships with Youth in Program Settings.*

46. R. D. Langhout, J. E. Rhodes, and L. Osborne, *Volunteer Mentoring with At-Risk Youth: Toward a Typology of Relationships.* (unpub.).

47. See, for example, S. F. Hamilton and M. A. Hamilton, "Mentoring programs: Promise and paradox," *Phi Delta Kappan* 73(7) (1992): 546–550; Sipe, "Mentoring adolescents," p. 16.

48. N. Darling, S. F. Hamilton, S. Niego, "Adolescents' relations with adults outside the family," in R. Montemeyor and G. R. Adams, eds., *Personal Relationships during Adolescence,* Advances in Adolescent Development: An Annual Book Series, 6 (Thousand Oaks, CA: Sage Publications, 1994), pp. 216–235.

49. Morrow and Styles, *Building Relationships with Youth in Program Settings.*

50. W. S. McClanahan, *Relationships in Career Mentoring Programs: Lessons Learned from the Hospital Youth Mentoring Program* (Philadelphia: Public/Private Ventures, 1998).

51. D. P. Keating, "Adolescent thinking," in S. S. Feldman and G. R. Elliott, eds., *At the Threshold: The Developing Adolescent* (Cambridge: Harvard University Press, 1990).

52. M. R. Beam, C. Chen, and E. Greenberger, "The nature of adolescents' relationships with their 'very important' nonparental adults," *American Journal of Community Psychology* (in press).

53. J. B. Grossman and A. Johnson, "Assessing the effectiveness of mentoring programs," in J. B. Grossman, ed., *Contemporary Issues in Mentoring* (Philadelphia: Public/Private Ventures 1998), pp. 48–65.

54. L. B. Hendry, W. Roberts, A. Glendinning, and J. C. Coleman, "Adolescents' perceptions of significant individuals in their lives," *Journal of Adolescence* 15(3) (1992): 255–270.

55. J. B. Grossman, J. Roffman, R. Reddy, and J. E. Rhodes. "Benchmarks of effective mentoring relationships" (unpub. ms., 2001).

56. The Helpfulness factor includes items 1–3, $\alpha = .81$; the Meeting Expectations factor includes items 4–6, $\alpha = .74$; the Negative Emotions factor includes items 7–12, $\alpha = .85$, and the Closeness factor includes items 1, 11, and 13–16, $\alpha = .81$. Many of these items were adapted for the outcome study from Wellborn and Connell's assessment package; see J. G. Wellborn and J. P. Connell, *Manual for the Rochester Assessment Package for Schools* (Rochester, NY: University of Rochester, 1987).

57. K. S. Rook. "Emotional health and positive versus negative social exchanges: A daily diary analysis," *Applied Developmental Science* 5(2) (2001): 86–97.

58. D. E. Orlinsky, K. Grawe, and B. K. Parks, "Process and outcome in psychotherapy: Noch einmal," in A. E. Bergin and S. L. Garfield, eds., *Handbook of Psychotherapy and Behavior Change*, 4th ed. (New York: John Wiley and Sons, 1994), pp. 270–376.

59. Ibid.

60. A. Bachelor and A. Horvath, "The therapeutic relationship," in M. A. Hubble, B. L. Duncan, and S. D. Miller, eds., *The Heart and Soul of Change: What Works in Therapy* (Washington, DC: American Psychological Association, 1999), pp. 133–178.

61. R. T. Dolan, D. B. Arnkoff, and C. R. Glass, "Client attachment style and the psychotherapist's interpersonal stance," *Psychotherapy* 30(3) (1993): 408–412.

62. Bachelor and Horvath, "The therapeutic relationship"; Orlinsky et al., "Process and outcome in psychotherapy."

63. Bachelor and Horvath, "The therapeutic relationship."

64. A. Bachelor, "Clients' perception of the therapeutic alliance: A qualitative analysis," *Journal of Counseling Psychology* 42 (1995): 323–337.

65. E. A. Ensher and S. E. Murphy, "Effects of race, gender, perceived similarity, and contact on mentor relationships," *Journal of Vocational Behavior* 50(3) (1997): 460–481.

66. M. Wierzbicki, and G. Pekarik, "A meta-analysis of psychotherapy dropout," *Professional Psychology—Research and Practice* 24(2) (May 1993): 190–195.

67. J. Hunsley, T. Aubry, C. Verstervelt, D. Vito, "Comparing therapist and client perspectives on reasons for psychotherapy termination," *Psychotherapy* 36(4) (Winter 1999): 380–388.

68. D. W. Winnicott, "Child analysis in the latency period," in *The Maturational Process and the Facilitative Environment* (New York: International Universities Press, 1958), p. 123; C. Siebold, "Termination: When the therapist leaves," *Clinical Social Work Journal* 19(2) (1991): 37.

69. Many of the recommendations for this discussion stemmed from two excellent guidebooks: J. Zaro, R. Barach, D. J. Nedelman, and I. S. Dreiblatt, *A Guide for Beginning Psychotherapists* (New York: Cambridge University Press); and D. Cangelosi, *Saying Goodbye in Child Psychotherapy: Planned, Unplanned, and Premature Endings* (Northvale, NJ: Jason Aronson, 1997).

70. Morrow and Styles, *Building Relationships with Youth in Program Settings*.

71. P. A. Dewald, "Forced termination of psychotherapy: The annually recurrent trauma," *Psychiatric Opinions*, January 1980, pp. 13–15.

72. J. Sandler, H. Kennedy, and R. L. Tyson, *The Technique Of Child Psychoanalysis: Discussions with Anna Freud* (Cambridge: Harvard University Press, 1980), p. 246.

73. For example, H. T. Reis and P. Shaver, "Intimacy as an interpersonal process," in S. Duck and D. F. Hay, eds., *Handbook of Personal Relationships: Theory, Research, and Interventions* (Chichester, England: Wiley, 1988), pp. 367–389.

74. P. Leach, *Babyhood* (New York: Alfred A. Knopf, 1989).

75. R. Coles, *The Call of Service: Witness to Idealism* (New York: Houghton Mifflin, 1994).

76. Z. Schachter-Shalomi and R. Miller, *From Age-ing to Sage-ing* (New York: Warner Books, 1994), pp. 200–202.

5. Mentoring in Perspective

1. M. Freedman, *The Kindness of Strangers: Adult Mentors, Urban Youth, and the New Volunteerism* (San Francisco: Jossey-Bass, 1993), p. 93. The phrase "fervor without infrastructure" has also been attributed to Mary Phillips, of the United Way of America who, in the early 1990s, called for fervor balanced with infrastructure in mentoring programs.

2. J. Roth, J. Brooks-Gunn, L. Murray, and W. Foster, "Promoting healthy adolescents: Synthesis of youth development program evaluations," *Journal of Research on Adolescence* 8(4) (1998): 423–459.

3. R. D. Putnam, *Bowling Alone: The Collapse And Revival Of American Community* (New York: Simon & Schuster, 2000).

4. S. Fordham and J. U. Ogbu, "Black students' school success: Coping with the 'burden of acting white,'" *Urban Review* 18(3) (1986): 176–206.

5. S. S. Luthar, "Vulnerability and resilience: A study of high-risk adolescents," *Child Development* 62(3) (1991): 600–616.

6. K. McCartney, and R. Rosenthal, "Effect size, practical importance, and social policy for children," *Child Development*. 71(1) (January–February, 2000): 173–180.

7. K. V. Morrow and M. B. Styles, *Building Relationships with Youth in Program Settings: A Study of Big Brothers/Big Sisters* (Philadelphia: Public/Private Ventures, 1995).

8. For example, the Relatedness Scale; see J. G. Wellborn and J. P. Connell, *Manual for the Rochester Assessment Package for Schools* (Rochester, NY: University of Rochester, 1987).

9. K. W. Fischer and C. Ayoub, "Analyzing development of working models of close relationships: Illustration with a case of vulnerability and violence," in G. G. Noam and K. W. Fischer, eds., *Development and Vulnerability in Close Relationships*, The Jean Piaget Symposium Series (Mahwah, NJ: Lawrence Erlbaum Associates, 1996), pp. 173–199.

10. J. B. Willett, J. D. Singer, and N. C. Martin, "The design and analysis of longitudinal studies of development and psychopathology in context: Statistical models and methodological recommendations," *Development and Psychopathology* 10 (1998): 395–426.

11. S. Kontos, "The role of continuity and context in children's relationships with nonparental adults," in R. C. Pianta, ed., *Beyond the Parent: The Role of Other Adults in Children's Lives*, New Directions in Child Development 57 (1992), pp. 81–108.

12. R. C. Pianta, *Enhancing Relationships between Children and Teachers* (Washington, DC: American Psychological Association, 1999), p. 188.

13. C. Herrera, *School-Based Mentoring: A First Look at Its Potential* (Philadelphia: Public/Private Ventures, 1999).

14. C. Herrera, C. L. Sipe, and W. S. McClanahan, with A. J. Arbreton and S. Pepper, *Mentoring School-Age Children: Relationship Development in Community-Based and School-Based Programs* (Philadelphia: Public/Private Ventures, 2000).

15. T. Curtis and K. Hansen-Schwoebel, *Big Brothers Big Sisters School-Based Mentoring: Evaluation Summary of Five Pilot Programs* (Philadelphia: Big Brothers Big Sisters of America, 1999).

16. R. H. Aseltine, M. Dupre, and P. Lamlein, "Mentoring as a drug prevention strategy: An evaluation of Across Ages," *Adolescent and Family Health* 1(1) (2000): 11–20.

17. Herrera, Sipe, and McClanahan, *Mentoring School-Age Children.*

18. Ibid.

19. J. E. Rhodes and A. A. Davis, "Supportive ties between nonparent adults and urban adolescent girls," in B. J. Leadbeater and N. Way, eds., *Urban Girls: Resisting Stereotypes, Creating Identities* (New York: New York University Press, 1996), pp. 213–249.

20. B. J. Hirsch, M. Mickus, and R. Boerger, *Ties to Influential Adults among Black and White* (in press).

21. R. W. Roeser, J. S. Eccles, and A. J. Sameroff, "Academic and emotional functioning in early adolescence: Longitudinal relations, patterns, and prediction by experience in middle school," *Development and Psychopathology* 10(2) (1998): 321–352.

22. J. Durlak and A. Wells, "Primary prevention mental health programs for children and adolescents: A meta-analytic review," *American Journal of Community Psychology* 25(2) (1997): 115–152.

23. R. C. Pianta, M. Stuhlman, and B. Hamre, "Enhancing youth development through relationships with nonparental adults: The value of student-teacher relationships and their implications for mentoring," in J. E. Rhodes, ed., *New Directions in Youth Development: Critical Perspectives on Youth Mentoring* (San Francisco: Jossey-Bass, in press).

24. Carnegie Council on Adolescent Development, *Turning Points: Preparing American Youth for the Twenty-First Century* (New York: Carnegie Corporation, 1989): p. 9.

25. J. D. Lempers and D. S. Clark-Lempers, "Young, middle, and late adolescents' comparisons of the functional importance of five significant relationships," *Journal of Youth and Adolescence* 21(1) (1992): 53–96.

26. M. Lynch and D. Cicchetti, "Children's relationships with adults and peers: An examination of elementary and junior high school students," *Journal of School Psychology* 35 (1997): 81–100.

27. J. Oakes, K. H. Quartz, S. Ryan, and Lipton, *Becoming Good American Schools: The Struggle for Civic Virtue in Education Reform* (San Francisco: Jossey-Bass Publishers), p. 155.

28. R. C. Pianta, *Enhancing Relationships between Children And Teachers* (Washington, DC: American Psychological Association, 1999).

29. Ibid.

30. R. W. Larson, "Toward a psychology of positive youth development," *American Psychologist* 55 (2000): 170–183.

31. S. B. Heath, *The Project of Learning from the Inner-City Youth Perspective*, New Directions for Child Development, 63 (San Francisco: Jossey-Bass, 1994), pp. 51–63; M. McLaughlin, M. Irby, and J. Langman, *Urban Sanctuaries: Neighborhood Organizations in the Lives and Future of Inner-City Youth* (San Francisco: Jossey-Bass, 1994).

32. M. Fine, L. Weis, C. Centrie and R. Roberts, "Educating beyond the borders of schooling," *Anthropology and Education* 31 (2000): 133.

33. J. G. Roffman, C. Suarez-Orozco, and J. E. Rhodes, "Facilitating positive development in immigrant youth: The role of mentors and community organizers," in D. F. Perkins, L. M. Borden, J. G. Keith, and F. A. Villarrurel, eds., *Positive Youth Development: Creating a Positive Tomorrow* (New York: Klewer Press, in press).

34. B. J. Hirsch, J. G. Roffman, N. L. Deutsch, C. Flynn, and M. E. Pagano, "Inner-city youth development programs: Strengthening programs for adolescent girls," *Journal of Early Adolescence* 20(2) (2000): 210–230.

35. M. B. Larner, L. Zippiroli, and R. E. Behrman, "When school is out: Analysis and recommendations," *Future of Children* 9(2) (1999): 4–20.

36. E. Seligson, "The policy climate for school-age child care," *Future of Children* 9(2) (1999): 145–159.

37. D. L. Vandell and L. Shumow, "After school child care programs," *Future of Children* 9(2) (1999): 64–80.

38. G. Walker and M. Freeman, "Social change one on one: The new mentoring movement," *American Prospect* 27 (1996): 75–81.

39. H. D. Trulear, *Faith-Based Institutions and High-Risk Youth* (Philadelphia: Public/Private Ventures, 2000).

40. T. D. Evans, F. T. Cullen, V. S. Burton, Jr., and R. G. Dunaway, "Religion, social bonds, and delinquency," *Deviant Behavior* 17(1) (January–March 1996): 43–70.

41. C. L. Sipe and S. Ma, *Community Change for Youth Development: Preliminary Report* (Philadelphia: Public/Private Ventures, 1999).

42. J. J. DiIulio, "Supporting black churches," *Brookings Review* 17 (1999): 3.

43. Two manuals are available to guide mentoring programs in the faith community: *Church-Based Mentoring: A Program Manual for Mentoring Ministries* (Alexandria, VA: The National Mentoring Partnership, 1999) and *Church Mentoring Network: A Program Manual for Linking and Supporting Mentoring Ministries* (Alexandria, VA: The National Mentoring Partnership, 1998).

44. K. McCartney and R. Rosenthal, "Effect size, practical importance, and social policy for children," *Child Development* 71 (2000): 173–180.

45. D. L. Fountain and A. Arbreton, "The costs of mentoring," in J. B. Grossman, ed., *Contemporary Issues in Mentoring* (Philadelphia: Public/Private Ventures, 1999).

46. Freedman, *The Kindness of Strangers*, p. 93.

47. R. Hunt, "Social entrepreneurs: The new philanthropists," *Wall Street Journal*, July 12, 2000, p. 1; A. Shanker, "Mentoring reconsidered," *American Federation of Teachers*, March 20, 1994.

48. E. Debold, L. M. Brown, S. Weseen, G. K. Brookins, "Cultivating hardiness zones for adolescent girls: A reconceptualization of resilience in relationships with caring adults," in N. G. Johnson and M. C. Roberts, eds., *Beyond Appearance: A New Look at Adolescent Girls* (Washington, DC: American Psychological Association, 1999), pp. 181–204; S. Mosle, "The vanity of volunteerism," *New York Times Magazine*, July 2, 2000, pp. 66–83.

49. R. D. Putnam, *Bowling Alone: The Collapse and Revival of American Community* (New York: Simon & Schuster, 2000).

50. Walker, "Social change one on one."

Acknowledgments

Carolyn Heilbrum once wrote that, “There is something all women like in an older, intelligent, assuaging female creature, and don’t let anyone tell you otherwise. Women don’t know how to define that comfort, because they find it so rarely, and because the word comfort seems to imply mindlessness . . . How many women older than you are there in your life, or have there ever been who have real power, whose minds you respect, and who are capable of being loved?” I am fortunate to have had two such women in my life, Sandra Oriel and Sandra Watanabe. Two extraordinary men have also served in this capacity, George Albee and Joseph McGrath. The force of these relationships has deeply influenced my thinking on the transforming potential of nonparent adult relationships.

A good part of the evidence and much of my understanding of mentoring were developed through a series of longitudinal research studies. I thus owe an enormous debt to the adolescents and mentors who have participated in the studies and whose voices and reports are at the heart of this book. I am also indebted to the colleagues, postdoctoral fellows, and graduate students who have collaborated with me over the years. Topping this list is Jean Baldwin Grossman, my collaborator in many of the studies reported in this book. I am thankful as well to Christina Gee, Jewell Hamilton-Leaks, Ranjini Reddy, and Jennifer Roffman. I acknowledge with gratitude the financial generosity of the William T. Grant Foundation, the National Institute of Child Health and Human Development, the Spencer Foundation, the Illinois Department of Human Services, and the Harvard University Graduate School of Education.

I have Frank Furstenberg to thank for suggesting that I write this book and for offering his editing and keen insights. Michael Aronson of Harvard University Press sponsored and guided this work from its inception, for which I am grateful. Many thanks go to Susan Wallace Boehmer, also of the Press, for improving this book through her skillful editing. I have relied on my community of family, friends, and colleagues for encouragement and support: Amanda Anderson, Jessica Ault, Tatiana Bertch, Dale Blythe, Paul Camic, Carol Gilligan, Rose Granowitz, Steve Granowitz, Barbara Linder, Sarah Mangelsdorf, Gil Noam, Carola Suarez-Orosco, Doug Russell, Pat Russell, Sabrina Shemesh, Renee Spencer, Deb Tolman, Niobe Way, and Kevin Wilson. I am especially indebted to Bart Hirsch, Julia Hough, Richard Lerner, Martha Mangelsdorf, Gail Manza, Robin Pringle, Nancy Rappaport, Juliet Schor, and Susan Weinberger for reading drafts and improving the book with their comments.

My sister, Nancy Rhodes McNamara, and my mother, Edith Rhodes, have buoyed me through life with their love and friendship. Molly Smith has given me real-world lessons on the joys and complexities of being a mentor. The lives of my children, Audrey, Ryan, and Thomas, are deeply intertwined with the writing of this book; I thank them for inspiring me, and Anadir Cappellari for keeping them healthy and happy while I wrote. Finally, but most important, I am inexpressibly grateful to my husband, Dane Wittrup, who bolstered me with his endless affection and wit.

Index

INDEX

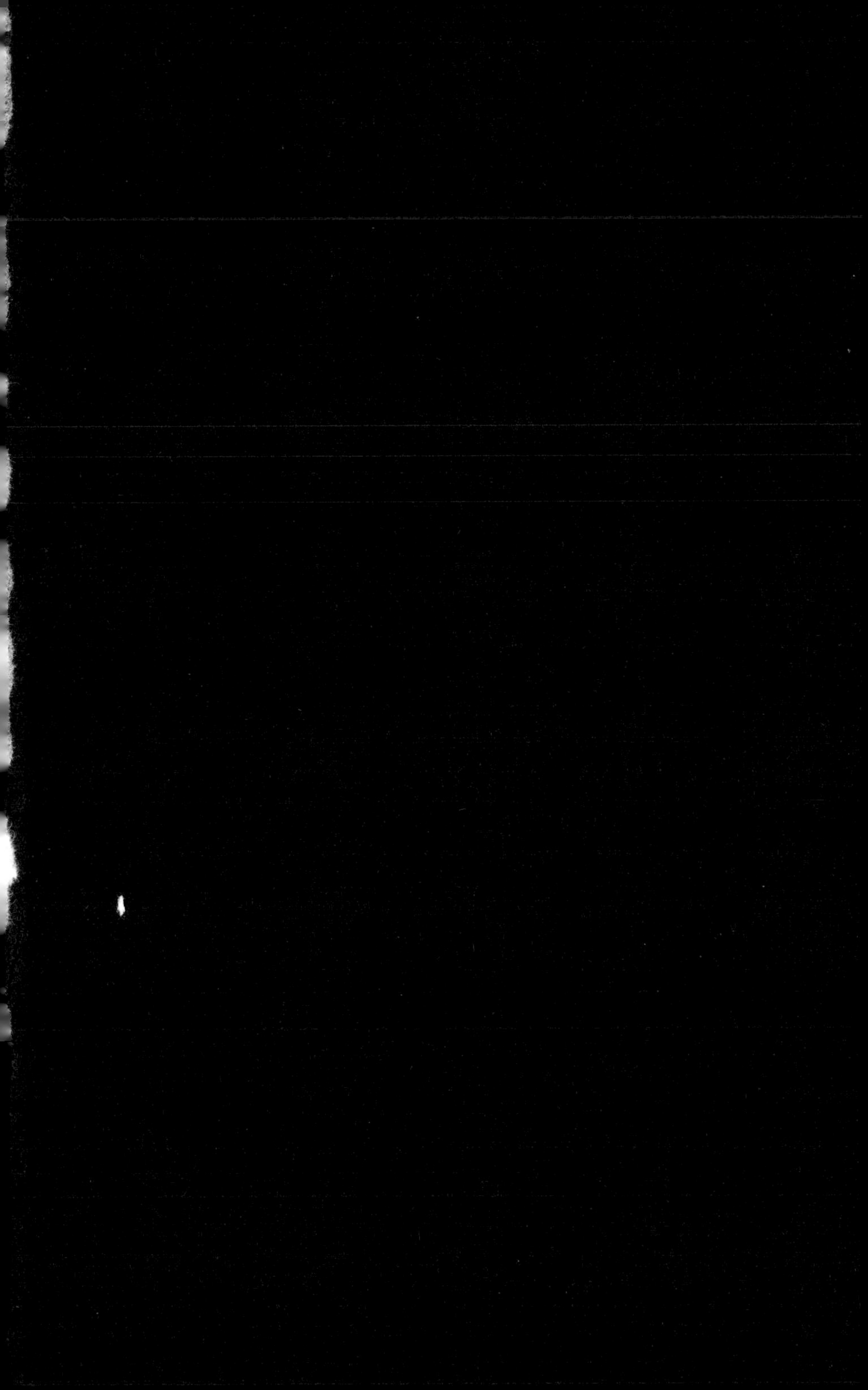